# ESSENTIAL CASES FOR FAMILY MEDICINE – FROM R1–R4: HOW TO PASS THE ARAB BOARDS

**Dr. Haider Ali, FRCGP, MBCHB, PGDIP Dermatology**
Consultant Family Medicine
Training Program Director, Family Medicine; Saudi German Hospital
Arab Board Examiner

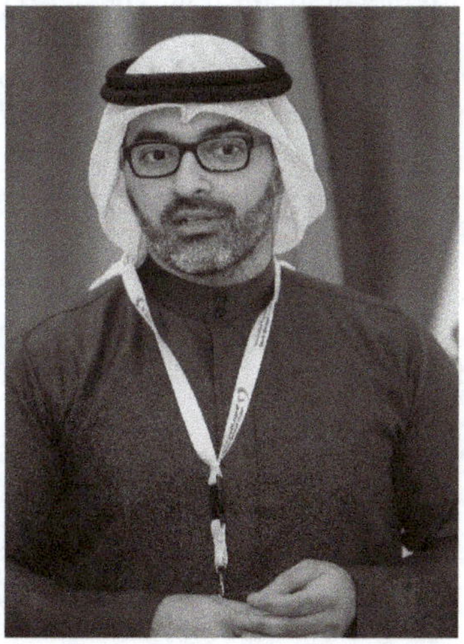

Mc Graw Hill

**Essential Cases for Family Medicine – From R1–R4: How to Pass the Arab Boards**



ISBN 978-1-265-78572-7
MHID 1-265-78572-4

**Notice**

Medicine is an ever-changing science. As new research and clinical experience broaden our knowledge, changes in treatment and drug therapy are required. The authors and the publisher of this work have checked with sources believed to be reliable in their efforts to provide information that is complete and generally in accord with the standards accepted at the time of publication. However, in view of the possibility of human error or changes in medical sciences, neither the authors nor the publisher nor any other party who has been involved in the preparation or publication of this work warrants that the information contained herein is in every respect accurate or complete, and they disclaim all responsibility for any errors or omissions, or for the results obtained from use of the information contained in this work. Readers are encouraged to confirm the information contained herein with other sources. For example and in particular, readers are advised to check the product information sheet included in the package of each drug they plan to administer to be certain that the information contained in this work is accurate and that changes have not been made in the recommended dose or in the contraindications for administration. This recommendation is of particular importance in connection with new or infrequently used drugs.

The editors were Michael Weitz and Kim J. Davis.
The production supervisor was Catherine Saggese.
The digital production manager was Steve Brown.
Project management was provided by Radhika Jolly of KnowledgeWorks Global Ltd.

Dear Resident:

It is with great hope and purpose that I present this collection of medical cases, carefully crafted to guide you along your training journey in family medicine. Each case is more than a clinical scenario – it is an opportunity to grow in knowledge, skill, and compassion.

As you progress through this book, may you be reminded of the profound impact you will have on your patients' lives.

The Qur'an beautifully emphasizes this truth:

*And whoever saves one [life] – it is as if he had saved all of humanity.*

وَمَنْ أَحْيَاهَا فَكَأَنَّمَا أَحْيَا ٱلنَّاسَ جَمِيعًا

**(Surah Al-Ma'idah, 5:32)**

This verse encapsulates the sacred purpose of your calling. In teaching and preparing you through this book, it is my sincere wish that you will be better equipped to fulfill this noble mission – to heal, to comfort, and to save lives.

May this book serve as a stepping stone in your journey to becoming not only skilled physicians but also compassionate caregivers, guided by the principles of empathy, excellence, and service to humanity.

With every case you solve, may you grow closer to fulfilling the immense responsibility and privilege of being a family medicine physician.

With hope for your success and unwavering belief in your potential,

**Dr. Haider Ali**

# Contents

# Preface

## What is the purpose of this book?

To support residents in their journey toward becoming skilled and compassionate family medicine specialists who provide comprehensive, patient-centred care that is evidence-based, high quality, and safe for everyone they serve in the UAE.

## How was this book developed and why?

I compiled this book because I believe practice consultations (aka mock consultations) are a powerful tool in family medicine training.

They offer residents the opportunity to practice diagnosing and managing both common and rare conditions in a safe and structured environment. This practice not only enhances clinical decision-making but also sharpens communication skills, builds confidence, and encourages a holistic, patient-centred approach to care.

By simulating diverse patient scenarios, residents can develop the skills needed to provide evidence-based, compassionate care in real-world practice.

In creating this book, residents at Saudi German Hospital Dubai, a family medicine resident from Sweden, and a medical student from Ajman Medical School on her family medicine rotation all contributed a case, reflecting their unique learning experiences. They have been actively engaging with the book, working through every case and participating in Balint-style discussions. These reflective discussions have enriched their understanding, fostered deeper insight into patient care, and supported their growth as future family physicians.

*With thanks to:*

*Dr. Namarig Murtada Amer Abdalla – Family Medicine Resident*
*Dr. Sawsan Abdelrahman Al-Darawi – Family Medicine Resident*
*Dr. Zainab Ali Ghaffori – Family Medicine Resident*
*Dr. Mohammad Alboareib – Paediatric Resident*
*Dr. Najwa Alani – Paediatric Resident*
*Dr. Noura Alali – Paediatric Resident*
*Dr. Marina Mingana – Family Medicine Resident (Sweden)*
*Dr. Najma Al Hamadi – Medical Intern*

A special thank you to Dr. Sabrin Ali, BDS UK, Content Editor, whose clinical insight and meticulous review of the cases ensured that they are both accurate and accessible for readers. Her commitment to clarity and user-friendliness has been invaluable.

I am equally grateful to Ms. Salama Alshebli, Creative Designer, for her vision and artistry in designing the book's cover. Her creativity has given the work a welcoming face that reflects the spirit of the content within.

## In what ways are practice consultations beneficial to residents?

1) **Exposure to a Variety of Cases**
   *Practice scenarios expose residents to diverse patient scenarios, including conditions they might not encounter frequently during clinical rotations.*
2) **Enhancing Clinical Decision-Making**
   By working through simulated cases, residents can refine their ability to gather relevant information, formulate differential diagnoses, and develop evidence-based management plans in a safe, supportive, and risk-free setting.

3) **Improving Communication Skills**
Family medicine requires effective communication with patients of all ages and backgrounds. Mock consultations help residents practice explaining diagnoses, discussing treatment options, and addressing patient concerns in a clear and empathetic manner.
4) **Building Confidence**
Having the opportunity to manage certain medical conditions with which the resident is not readily familiar will help boost their confidence in their clinical abilities.
5) **Feedback and Reflection**
Our mock consultations/simulated cases always include structured feedback from supervisors or peers, helping residents identify areas for improvement and learn from their mistakes without compromising patient safety. This is done in the Calgary Cambridge method without judgement and always with support.
6) **Holistic Approach to Patient Care**
These simulations often emphasise patient-centred care, teaching residents to consider the physical, emotional, and social aspects of a patient's health, which is one of the fundamental aspects of family medicine.

## Tips and Tricks for Doctors – How to Make Use of Communication

1) *Use positive and reassuring language*
Say, "Let me have a thorough look at your knee/throat/painful joint," rather than "Let me have a quick look."
Using words like "thorough" shows patients that you are taking their concerns seriously and giving them your full attention. In contrast, "quick" can make patients feel dismissed or that their issue is not important.
2) *Mirroring – a communication hack*
When presented with a patient's complaint: "Doc, I've had a cough for 3 weeks now."
Say: "You've had a cough for 3 weeks? Gosh, that sounds terrible."
Mirroring can build rapport and help the patient feel understood and comfortable, fostering trust.
3) *Use active listening*
Maintain eye contact, nod, and provide verbal affirmations like "I understand" or "Tell me more," as this emphasises your candid interest in the patient's issue/medical history, which further develops rapport.
4) *Use open-ended questions*
"Can you tell me more about how this pain started?"
This encourages patients to give you further, often important information that will assist in data gathering and eventually diagnosis.
5) *Avoid medical jargon*
Instead of "You might have a myocardial infarction," say, "It looks like you might be having a heart attack."
Using clear and simple language (aka layman's terms) ensures that patients fully understand their condition and treatment options.
6) *Address ICE (Ideas, Concerns, and Expectations)*

| | |
|---|---|
| Ideas: | "What do you think might be causing this?" |
| Concerns: | "Is there anything you're particularly worried about?" |
| Expectations: | "What were you hoping I would do for you today?" |

The use of ICE is known to help uncover potential hidden agendas and will guide you as a health care professional to provide reassurance, education, and help build trust, which equates to patient-centred care.
7) *Acknowledge and validate feelings – pick up on cues*
"It's completely understandable to feel anxious about this."
Validating emotions makes the patient feel heard and respected, which strengthens the doctor–patient relationship.

8) *Consider ending the consultation with a summary and invite questions:*
"To summarise, we've discussed [key points]."
"Does that make sense? Is there anything else you'd like to ask?"
Summarising ensures the patient understands the plan and invites them to clarify or raise additional concerns which can further support rapport and address any further concerns promptly and safely.

**Dr. Haider Ali, FRCGP, MBCHB, PGDIP Dermatology**
Training Program Director, Family Medicine
Family Medicine Consultant
Fellow Royal College General Practitioners

CASE 1

# Traveller's Diarrhoea

## Doctor's Notes

*Patient Details:*

- **Name:** Ahmed Mansour
- **Age:** 34
- **Occupation:** IT Consultant
- **Presenting Complaint:** Diarrhoea after recent travel
- **Setting:** Family Medicine Clinic

## PATIENT'S SIMULATED SCRIPT:

### Opening Statement:

"Doctor, I've been having diarrhoea since I returned from my trip to India."

## HISTORY:

- **Onset:** Began 3 days ago, shortly after returning from a 2-week business trip to India.
- **Frequency:** Passing loose stools six to eight times daily.
- **Consistency:** Watery, no blood or mucus observed.
- **Associated Symptoms:** Mild abdominal cramps, fatigue, occasional nausea but no vomiting or fever.
- **Hydration Status:** Feels thirsty and lightheaded; reduced frequency of urination.
- **Dietary History:** Consumed meals at local restaurants and street food during the trip.
- **Travel History:** No pre-travel vaccinations for typhoid or hepatitis A. Stayed in urban areas, drank bottled water but consumed drinks with ice.
- **Past Episodes:** No similar previous episodes.

## DRUG HISTORY:

- **Regular Medications:** None.
- **Allergies:** None known.
- **Recent Medications:** Took loperamide once yesterday, which slightly reduced stool frequency. No antibiotics.

## FAMILY HISTORY:

- No family history of gastrointestinal diseases or chronic illnesses.

## IDEAS, CONCERNS, EXPECTATIONS:

- **Ideas:** Thinks he might have got stomach flu, as with a bad cold previously he has had similar previously.
- **Concerns:** Worried it could be a serious infection that might worsen or spread.
- **Expectations:** Looking for medication to stop the diarrhoea and advice on how to prevent similar issues in the future.

## ON EXAMINATION:

- **General Appearance:** Alert but appears slightly fatigued.
- **Vitals:** BP 110/70 mmHg, HR 90 bpm (regular), temperature 37.2°C.
- **Hydration Status:** Mild dehydration (dry mucous membranes, delayed skin turgor).
- **Abdominal Examination:** Mild tenderness in the lower abdomen, no guarding or rigidity, bowel sounds present and hyperactive.

## INVESTIGATIONS:

### Stool Analysis Report:

*Macroscopic Examination*

- **Colour:** Brown
- **Consistency:** Soft
- **Blood:** Absent
- **Mucus:** Absent

*Microscopic Examination*

- **White Blood Cells (WBC):** Moderate
- **Red Blood Cells (RBC):** None
- **Parasites:** None identified
- **Ova and Cysts:** Absent

*Culture and Sensitivity*

**Organism Identified:** *Escherichia coli* – Pathogenic strain detected (e.g., Enterotoxigenic *E. coli* [ETEC] or Shiga toxin–producing *E. coli* [STEC]).

## WHAT IS THE DIAGNOSIS?

**Traveller's Diarrhoea** – likely bacterial.

Traveller's diarrhoea is a common stomach condition that many people experience while visiting new places. It often occurs after consuming food or water contaminated with germs, particularly in regions where food safety practices may differ. Symptoms typically include loose stools, stomach cramps, bloating, and sometimes nausea. Most cases resolve on their own within a few days with rest, plenty of fluids, and over-the-counter medications. To reduce the risk, it's best to drink bottled water, avoid raw or undercooked foods, and maintain good hygiene.

## HOW WOULD YOU MANAGE THIS PATIENT?

### Management Options:

1. **Hydration:** Emphasize oral rehydration using oral rehydration salts (ORS) or homemade solutions (water with salt and sugar).
2. **Dietary Advice:** Recommend avoiding solid foods until symptoms improve, then resume a bland diet (e.g., rice, bananas, toast).
3. **Medications:**
   - Continue loperamide for symptom relief with caution on overuse.
   - Prescribe a short course of antibiotics (e.g., azithromycin) if symptoms persist or worsen.
4. **Red Flags:** Advise immediate medical attention if symptoms like fever, bloody stools, or persistent diarrhoea beyond 7 days occur.

**What factors in this case suggest a bacterial cause of traveller's diarrhoea rather than a viral or parasitic one?**

Moderate WBCs in stool, absence of blood/mucus (suggesting enterotoxigenic rather than invasive), recent travel to endemic area, and identification of pathogenic *E. coli* on stool culture.

**What advice would you give the patient to reduce the risk of traveller's diarrhoea in future trips?**

Drink bottled or properly treated water; avoid ice, raw fruits/vegetables unless peeled; eat freshly cooked food; consider pre-travel vaccines (e.g., typhoid, hepatitis A)

**When would you consider referring this patient for further evaluation or hospital admission?**

If there is high fever, bloody diarrhoea, signs of severe dehydration, persistent symptoms beyond 7 days, or inability to tolerate oral fluids.

## FOLLOW-UP:

- Schedule a follow-up visit in 1 week to confirm symptom resolution.

## SAFETY NETTING:

- Educate about warning signs such as high fever, severe abdominal pain, inability to keep fluids down, and signs of severe dehydration.
- Stress the importance of hygiene measures (e.g., regular handwashing, careful food handling) to prevent the spread of infection.

CASE 2

# Smoking Cessation

## Doctor's Notes

*Patient Details:*

- **Name:** Khalid Al-Mansouri
- **Age:** 45
- **Occupation:** Accountant
- **Presenting Complaint:** Request for help with quitting smoking
- **Setting:** Family Medicine Clinic

## PATIENT'S SIMULATED SCRIPT:

### Opening Statement:

"Doctor, I've been smoking for years, and I really want to quit now."

## HISTORY:

- **Smoking History:**
  - Smokes 20 cigarettes daily for the past 25 years (20-pack-year history).
  - Has attempted to quit twice in the past, but relapsed within a few weeks.
  - Triggers for smoking include stress at work and social gatherings.
- **Motivation to Quit:** Strong motivation due to health concerns and a recent family history of heart disease.
- **Associated Symptoms:** Occasional morning cough but no shortness of breath, chest pain, or other respiratory symptoms.
- **Previous Quit Methods:** Tried nicotine gum and reducing the number of cigarettes, both without success.
- **Other Lifestyle Factors:** No regular exercise; consumes two to three cups of coffee daily, occasionally smokes shisha during social events.

## DRUG HISTORY:

- **Regular Medications:** None.
- **Allergies:** None known.
- **Recent Medications:** None related to smoking cessation.

## FAMILY HISTORY:

- Father passed away from a heart attack at age 60; was also a heavy smoker.
- No family history of cancer or chronic lung diseases.

## IDEAS, CONCERNS, EXPECTATIONS:

- **Ideas:** Believes smoking is harming his health, especially with his family history of heart disease. Has been advised numerous times to quit and feels this is the right time.
- **Concerns:** Worried about long-term damage from smoking and fears withdrawal symptoms during quitting. Is worried he'll be grumpy and mean.
- **Expectations:** Seeking guidance on effective strategies to quit and hoping for support to manage cravings. Hopes the doctor can reduce any bad symptoms.

## ON EXAMINATION:

- **General Appearance:** Well-groomed and cooperative.
- **Vitals:** BP 130/85 mmHg, HR 88 bpm, respiratory rate 16/min, temperature 36.8°C.
- **Respiratory Examination:** Clear lung fields with normal breath sounds, no wheezing or crackles.
- **Cardiovascular Examination:** Heart sounds normal, no murmurs.
- Consider asking for carbon monoxide levels at the start of the smoking cessation program and throughout.

## WHAT IS THE DIAGNOSIS?

**Chronic Tobacco Dependence** with high motivation to quit.

Tobacco dependence is a condition where the body and mind become reliant on nicotine, the addictive substance in tobacco. Over time, this leads to cravings and withdrawal symptoms when not smoking, making it difficult to quit. Regular use can harm nearly every organ, increasing the risk of serious health issues like lung disease, heart problems, and cancer. Treatment often involves counselling, nicotine replacement products, or medications to manage cravings and support quitting.

## HOW WOULD YOU MANAGE THIS PATIENT?

1. **Counselling and Behavioural Support:**
   - Explore triggers and coping strategies to handle stress and cravings.
   - Provide information on the health benefits of quitting smoking.
   - Discuss setting a quit date and preparing for withdrawal symptoms.
2. **Pharmacotherapy:**
   - Offer nicotine replacement therapy (e.g., patches, gum, or lozenges) tailored to the patient's needs.
   - Discuss prescription medications such as varenicline or bupropion as options if nicotine replacement alone is insufficient.
3. **Lifestyle Modifications:**
   - Encourage regular physical activity to reduce stress and improve mood.
   - Advise reducing caffeine intake, as quitting smoking may enhance caffeine sensitivity.

4. **Follow-up Support:**
   - Schedule regular follow-up appointments for monitoring and encouragement.
   - Refer to smoking cessation support groups if available.

## HOW DO VARENICLINE AND BUPROPION WORK?

### Varenicline (Champix):

Reduces cravings and withdrawal symptoms by partially stimulating nicotine receptors in the brain while blocking the pleasurable effects of nicotine from cigarettes.

Take 1–2 weeks prior to deciding on the date you wish to stop smoking ("quit date").

Increase the dose gradually with an average treatment of 12 weeks.

Caution with using with patients with depression/anxiety, as it is reported to affect mood, although this is uncommon.

### Bupropion (Zyban):

Technically this medication is an antidepressant that also reduces nicotine cravings and withdrawal symptoms through its action on dopamine and norepinephrine.

Take 1–2 weeks prior to deciding on the date you wish to stop smoking ("quit date").

Treatment duration is 7–12 weeks.

**Caution with patients with epilepsy, as can increase seizure risk.**

Varenicline is considered the first-line treatment for patients with intense cravings, and Bupropion is ideal for those requiring mood management in addition to wanting to quit smoking.

## FOLLOW-UP:

- Regular follow-ups to support compliance and review mental health specially if on Varenicline.

## SAFETY NETTING:

- Educate about withdrawal symptoms (e.g., irritability, cravings, difficulty concentrating) and reassure that these are temporary.
- Encourage contacting the clinic if experiencing severe mood changes, relapse, or other concerns.
- Emphasize the importance of reaching out for support rather than giving up if a relapse occurs.

CASE 3

# Osteoporosis

## Doctor's Notes

*Patient Details:*

- **Name:** Layla Al-Shehri
- **Age:** 65
- **Occupation:** Retired teacher
- **Presenting Complaint:** Review of DEXA scan results
- **Setting:** Family Medicine Clinic

## PATIENT'S SIMULATED SCRIPT:

### Opening Statement:

"Doctor, I'm here to discuss my bone scan results."

## HISTORY:

- **Background:**
  - History of mild back pain over the last few months but no history of fractures.
  - Menopause at age 50, no hormone replacement therapy.
  - Minimal physical activity; spends most of her time indoors.
  - Diet low in calcium; does not consume dairy regularly.
- **DEXA Scan Results:**
  - T-score: −2.8 at the lumbar spine, **consistent with osteoporosis**.
  - T-score: −2.1 at the hip, **consistent with osteopenia**.
- **Risk Factors:**
  - Family history of osteoporosis (mother had a hip fracture at 70).
  - Long-term use of proton pump inhibitors for reflux.
- **Impact on Life:** No significant limitations in daily activities but concerned about her risk of fractures.

## DRUG HISTORY:

- **Regular Medications:** Omeprazole 20 mg daily for GERD, multivitamin occasionally.
- **Allergies:** None known.
- **Recent Medications:** None specific for bone health.

## FAMILY HISTORY:

- Mother had osteoporosis and sustained a hip fracture at age 70.
- No family history of other significant chronic diseases.

## IDEAS, CONCERNS, EXPECTATIONS:

- **Ideas:** Believes the scan indicates she must have wear and tear arthritis.
- **Concerns:** Worried that she will end up very mobility restricted and on crutches soon.
- **Expectations:** Looking for advice on how to avoid that, maybe with some medications or injections.

## ON EXAMINATION:

- **General Appearance:** Alert, well-nourished, no acute distress.
- **Vitals:** BP 125/80 mmHg, HR 75 bpm, temperature 36.7°C.
- **Musculoskeletal Examination:**
    - Normal posture and gait.
    - No tenderness or deformities in the spine or hips.
    - Full range of motion in joints.

## WHAT IS THE DIAGNOSIS?

**Osteoporosis** based on DEXA scan results and clinical risk factors.

Osteoporosis is a bone disease characterized by decreased bone density and strength, making bones fragile and more susceptible to fractures. It occurs when bone resorption outpaces bone formation, leading to porous and brittle bones. Risk factors include aging, hormonal changes (especially in postmenopausal women), poor nutrition, sedentary lifestyle, and genetic predisposition. Common fracture sites include the hip, spine, and wrist. Prevention and management involve calcium and vitamin D intake, weight-bearing exercise, and medications like bisphosphonates.

## HOW WOULD YOU MANAGE THIS PATIENT?

1. **Lifestyle Modifications:**
    - Encourage weight-bearing exercises (e.g., walking, light resistance training) to strengthen bones.
    - Advise a diet rich in calcium (e.g., leafy greens, fortified foods) and vitamin D.
    - Recommend spending time outdoors for natural vitamin D synthesis.
2. **Pharmacotherapy:**
    - Prescribe a bisphosphonate (e.g., alendronate 70 mg once weekly) to improve bone density.
    - Supplement with calcium (1200 mg daily) and vitamin D3 (800–1000 IU daily).
    - Review and consider alternatives to long-term omeprazole use to reduce further bone loss.
3. **Education and Prevention:**
    - Teach fall prevention strategies: adequate lighting, removing tripping hazards, and using assistive devices if needed.
    - Discuss the importance of medication adherence and regular follow-up for monitoring bone density.

**What factors put this patient at increased risk for osteoporosis-related fractures?**

Postmenopausal status, low physical activity, poor calcium intake, maternal history of hip fracture, long-term PPI use, low lumbar spine T-score (−2.8).

**What is the role of bisphosphonates in osteoporosis management, and what key counselling points should be provided?**

Bisphosphonates inhibit bone resorption and reduce fracture risk. Counsel to take on an empty stomach with water, stay upright for 30 minutes, and report any GI symptoms or jaw pain (rare osteonecrosis).

**How would you monitor this patient after initiating treatment for osteoporosis?**

Repeat DEXA scan in 1–2 years, assess adherence and side effects, monitor calcium/vitamin D status, and reassess fracture risk (e.g., FRAX score).

## FOLLOW-UP:

- Arrange a follow-up visit in 3–6 months to assess adherence to treatment and lifestyle changes.
- Repeat DEXA scan in 1–2 years to evaluate treatment effectiveness.

## SAFETY NETTING:

- Advise immediate consultation if she experiences new or worsening back pain, height loss, or signs of fractures.
- Educate on potential side effects of bisphosphonates (e.g., gastrointestinal discomfort) and when to seek advice.

CASE

# 4

# *Helicobacter pylori*

## Doctor's Notes

*Patient Details:*

- **Name:** Fatima Al-Harbi
- **Age:** 38
- **Occupation:** Teacher
- **Presenting Complaint:** Follow-up to discuss results of a breath test for stomach issues
- **Setting:** Family Medicine Clinic

## PATIENT'S SIMULATED SCRIPT:

### Opening Statement:

"Doctor, I'm here to find out the results of my stomach test."

## HISTORY:

- **Presenting Symptoms:**
  - Recurrent upper abdominal discomfort for the past 6 months, described as a burning sensation.
  - Symptoms worse on an empty stomach and occasionally wake her at night.
  - No associated weight loss, vomiting, or blood in stool.
  - Occasional bloating and nausea, particularly after heavy meals.
- **Aggravating Factors:** Spicy foods and stress.
- **Relieving Factors:** Antacids provide temporary relief.
- **Impact on Life:** Symptoms affect her concentration at work and disrupt her sleep occasionally.

## DRUG HISTORY:

- **Regular Medications:** Over-the-counter antacids as needed (uses three to four times a week).
- **Allergies:** None known.
- **Recent Medications:** Non-specific for stomach issues.

## FAMILY HISTORY:

- Father has a history of peptic ulcer disease, treated successfully.
- No family history of gastric cancer or other gastrointestinal conditions.

## IDEAS, CONCERNS, EXPECTATIONS:

- **Ideas:** Wonders if her symptoms are related to stress or something she's eating.
- **Concerns:** Worried it would get worse and she may need time off work. She's already behind with work due to upcoming exams and marking.
- **Expectations:** Hoping for a clear explanation of the cause and effective treatment options.

## ON EXAMINATION:

- **General Appearance:** Alert and well-nourished.
- **Vitals:** BP 120/75 mmHg, HR 78 bpm, temperature 36.8°C.
- **Abdominal Examination:**
  - Soft and non-distended.
  - Mild epigastric tenderness on deep palpation.
  - No guarding, rebound tenderness, or palpable masses.
- **Positive urea breath test.**

## WHAT IS THE DIAGNOSIS?

***Helicobacter Pylori* Infection** confirmed by positive urea breath test.

*H. pylori* is a type of bacteria that lives in the stomach and can cause problems like stomach ulcers, gastritis (inflammation of the stomach lining), and even increase the risk of stomach cancer. It survives in the stomach's acidic environment by producing a special enzyme (urease) that helps neutralize stomach acid. People usually get it through contaminated food, water, or close contact with an infected person.

Many people have *H. pylori* without symptoms, but if it causes issues, doctors diagnose it with breath, stool, or blood tests. Treatment usually involves a mix of antibiotics and acid-reducing medications to get rid of the infection.

## HOW WOULD YOU MANAGE THIS PATIENT?

1. **Education:**
   - Explain the diagnosis of *H. pylori* infection and its role in causing symptoms like gastritis or peptic ulcer disease.
   - Reassure that it is treatable and curable in most cases.
2. **Eradication Therapy:**
   - Prescribe a 14-day course of triple therapy: a proton pump inhibitor (e.g., omeprazole 20 mg twice daily) and two antibiotics (e.g., amoxicillin 1 g twice daily and clarithromycin 500 mg twice daily).
   - Discuss possible side effects (e.g., nausea, diarrhoea) and the importance of completing the full course.
3. **Lifestyle and Dietary Advice:**
   - Avoid triggers such as spicy foods, caffeine, and NSAIDs.
   - Manage stress through relaxation techniques or counselling if necessary.
   - Encourage smaller, more frequent meals.
4. **Follow-up Plan:**
   - Arrange a follow-up appointment in 4–6 weeks after completing therapy to assess symptom resolution.
   - Offer a repeat breath test or stool antigen test to confirm eradication if clinically indicated.

**Why is triple therapy recommended for treating *H. pylori*, and what are the key components?**

Triple therapy combines a proton pump inhibitor with two antibiotics (usually amoxicillin and clarithromycin) to eradicate the bacteria and promote mucosal healing.

**What advice should you give to ensure successful *H. pylori* eradication?**

Emphasize adherence to the full 14-day course, timing of doses, and managing side effects; avoid alcohol and NSAIDs during treatment.

**When and how should eradication of *H. pylori* be confirmed?**

If symptoms persist or in high-risk cases, confirm with a urea breath test or stool antigen test at least 4 weeks after completing therapy.

## SAFETY NETTING:

- Advise seeking immediate medical attention for any alarming symptoms, such as vomiting blood, black stools, severe abdominal pain, or unexplained weight loss.
- Encourage returning to the clinic if symptoms persist or worsen despite treatment.

CASE 5

# Needle Stick Injury

## Doctor's Notes

*Patient Details:*

- **Name:** Ahmed Al-Farsi
- **Age:** 32
- **Occupation:** General Practitioner
- **Presenting Complaint:** Needle stick injury sustained during a patient procedure
- **Setting:** Family Medicine Clinic

## PATIENT'S SIMULATED SCRIPT:

### Opening Statement:

"Doctor, I accidentally pricked myself with a needle during a procedure on a patient, and I'm really worried."

## HISTORY:

- **Injury Details:**
  - Occurred while suturing a patient known to be a chronic HBV carrier.
  - The needle was used for suturing and had been exposed to the patient's blood.
  - Incident occurred approximately 1 hour ago.
  - Immediate first aid was performed: washed with soap and water, no antiseptic used.
- **Vaccination History:**
  - Received full hepatitis B vaccination series during medical school.
  - Unsure of last antibody titre test or booster.
- **Symptoms Post-Injury:**
  - No symptoms at present, no visible inflammation or signs of infection at the injury site.

## DRUG HISTORY:

- **Regular Medications:** None.
- **Allergies:** None known.
- **Recent Medications:** None specific.

## FAMILY HISTORY:

- No family history of hepatitis or other chronic infections.
- General good health in the family.

## IDEAS, CONCERNS, EXPECTATIONS:

- **Ideas:** Has been told that although unlikely, he should get checked out in case he catches an infection from the patient.
- **Concerns:** Highly anxious about contracting HBV despite vaccination and about potential implications for his health and work.
- **Expectations:** Expects immediate testing and guidance on post-exposure prophylaxis (PEP).

## ON EXAMINATION:

- **General Appearance:** Alert and anxious but otherwise healthy.
- **Vitals:** BP 118/76 mmHg, HR 80 bpm, temperature 36.7°C.
- **Examination of Injury Site:**
  - Small puncture wound on the right index finger.
  - No signs of bleeding, redness, or swelling.

## WHAT IS THE DIAGNOSIS?

**Needle Stick Injury (NSI)** with potential exposure to HBV from a chronic carrier patient.

## HOW WOULD YOU MANAGE THIS PATIENT?

1. **Immediate Steps:**
   - Reassure the patient and provide psychological support.
   - Perform baseline serology testing:
     - Dr. Ahmed: HBsAg, anti-HBs, anti-HBc, anti-HCV, HIV serology.
     - Patient (source): Confirm HBV status, HCV, and HIV status if not already known.
2. **PEP:**
   - If anti-HBs titres are ≥10 mIU/mL:
     - Reassure that no further action is needed for HBV prophylaxis.
   - If anti-HBs titres are <10 mIU/mL:
     - Administer hepatitis B immunoglobulin (HBIG) and a booster dose of hepatitis B vaccine within 24 hours.
3. **Further Follow-up:**
   - Arrange repeat serology tests at 6 weeks, 3 months, and 6 months for HBV, HCV, and HIV.
   - Emphasize avoiding blood donation or high-risk activities until follow-up is complete.
4. **Education:**
   - Discuss safe practices to minimize future NSI risks.
   - Reinforce the importance of regular updates to vaccination and antibody titres.

**What factors determine the need for HBV post-exposure prophylaxis in this case?**

The exposed person's anti-HBs titre and the source patient's HBV status. If anti-HBs <10 mIU/mL and source is HBsAg positive, HBIG positive vaccine booster is required.

**What baseline and follow-up tests are appropriate for this exposure?**

Baseline: HBsAg, anti-HBs, anti-HBc, anti-HCV, HIV. Follow-up at 6 weeks, 3 months, and 6 months to monitor seroconversion.

**What immediate counselling should be given regarding infection risk and work precautions?**

Reassure that transmission risk is low if vaccinated; avoid blood donation and high-risk exposures until follow-up is complete; advise on proper sharps disposal and incident reporting.

## SAFETY NETTING:

- Advise seeking urgent medical attention for fever, jaundice, or other concerning symptoms.
- Provide contact details for immediate consultation if he develops symptoms or has further questions.

CASE 6

# Coeliac Disease

## Doctor's Notes

*Patient Details:*

- **Name:** Yasser Al-Khalidi
- **Age:** 29
- **Occupation:** Engineer
- **Presenting Complaint:** Chronic diarrhoea and follow-up on recent lab test results
- **Setting:** Family Medicine Clinic

## PATIENT'S SIMULATED SCRIPT:

### Opening Statement:

"Doctor, I'm here to discuss the results of my tests. I've still been having diarrhoea, and it's been quite frustrating."

## HISTORY:

- **Presenting Symptoms:**
  - Diarrhoea for the past 4–5 months, with three to four loose stools daily.
  - Associated symptoms: bloating, occasional abdominal discomfort, and fatigue.
  - No blood in stool or nocturnal diarrhoea.
  - No significant weight loss but feels more tired than usual.
- **Dietary History:**
  - Eats a varied diet including bread, pasta, and other gluten-containing foods daily.
- **Impact on Life:**
  - Increased fatigue has affected work performance.
  - Socially anxious about frequent trips to the bathroom.

## DRUG HISTORY:

- **Regular Medications:** None.
- **Allergies:** None known.
- **Recent Medications:** Occasionally uses over-the-counter antidiarrhoeals, which provide limited relief.

## FAMILY HISTORY:

- Mother diagnosed with hypothyroidism.
- Two paternal aunts with diabetes.
- No family history of gastrointestinal conditions.

## IDEAS, CONCERNS, EXPECTATIONS:

- **Ideas:** Thinks it might be related to something he's eating but unsure what.
- **Concerns:** Worried about a serious underlying condition and long-term effects of persistent diarrhoea.
- **Expectations:** Wants clarity on the test results and a solution to improve his symptoms.

## ON EXAMINATION:

- **General Appearance:** Looks slightly pale but otherwise well.
- **Vitals:** BP 118/74 mmHg, HR 76 bpm, temperature 36.9°C.
- **Abdominal Examination:**
  - Soft and non-tender.
  - No masses or organomegaly.
  - Normal bowel sounds.

| Parameter | Result | Reference Range |
|---|---|---|
| Haemoglobin (Hb) | 9.0 g/dL | 12.0–15.5 g/dL (F) |
| Haematocrit (Hct) | 28.0% | 36.0–45.0% (F) |
| Red Blood Cell Count (RBC) | 4.0 × $10^6$/μL | 4.1–5.1 × $10^6$/μL (F) |
| Mean Corpuscular Volume (MCV) | 68 fL | 80–100 fL |
| Mean Corpuscular Haemoglobin (MCH) | 21 pg | 27–33 pg |
| Mean Corpuscular Haemoglobin Concentration (MCHC) | 30 g/dL | 32–36 g/dL |
| Red Cell Distribution Width (RDW) | 16.5% | 11.5–14.5% |
| White Blood Cell Count (WBC) | 6.5 × $10^3$/μL | 4.5–11.0 × $10^3$/μL |
| Platelet Count | 450 × $10^3$/μL | 150–400 × $10^3$/μL |

## WHAT IS THE DIAGNOSIS?

- **Iron Deficiency Anaemia** (based on iron panel results).
- **Coeliac Disease** (based on positive coeliac serology).

Coeliac disease is a condition where the immune system reacts abnormally to gluten, a protein found in wheat, barley, and rye. When people with coeliac disease eat gluten, their immune system attacks the lining of the small intestine, causing damage that makes it harder to absorb nutrients. This can lead to symptoms like diarrhoea, bloating, stomach pain, fatigue, and weight loss. If left untreated, it can cause serious health problems, including malnutrition and osteoporosis. The only treatment is a strict gluten-free diet, which helps heal the intestine and prevent further damage.

## HOW WOULD YOU MANAGE THIS PATIENT?

1. **Discussion:**
   - Explain the diagnosis of coeliac disease and its association with chronic diarrhoea and iron deficiency anaemia.
   - Emphasize the autoimmune nature of the condition and the need for lifelong adherence to a gluten-free diet.
2. **Dietary Advice:**
   - Refer to a dietitian for guidance on a strict gluten-free diet.
   - Provide resources on identifying gluten-containing foods and gluten-free alternatives.
   - Discuss potential challenges and ways to avoid cross-contamination.
3. **Iron Supplementation:**
   - Start oral iron supplementation
   - Reassess iron levels in 2–3 months.
4. **Further Investigations:**
   - Arrange for a referral to gastroenterology for confirmation via endoscopic biopsy of the small intestine.
   - Screen for other nutritional deficiencies (e.g., vitamin D, calcium, folate, $B_{12}$).
5. **Supportive Measures:**
   - Address concerns about lifestyle adjustments and offer psychological support if needed.

**What other clinical findings in this case support the diagnosis of coeliac disease?**

Chronic diarrhoea, fatigue, bloating, positive coeliac serology, and microcytic anaemia (Hb 9.0 g/dL, MCV 68 fL) suggest malabsorption due to coeliac disease.

**Why is a gluten-free diet essential in coeliac disease, and what challenges might the patient face?**

A gluten-free diet is the only effective treatment to prevent intestinal damage and complications. Challenges include hidden gluten in processed foods, social dining, and cross-contamination.

**What additional health checks should be considered in a newly diagnosed coeliac patient?**

Screen for other autoimmune conditions (e.g., thyroid disease), nutritional deficiencies (iron, $B_{12}$, vitamin D, calcium), and recommend bone density assessment if indicated.

## FOLLOW-UP:

- Schedule a follow-up appointment in 6–8 weeks to assess symptom improvement and adherence to the gluten-free diet.
- Monitor iron levels and haemoglobin to evaluate response to supplementation.

## SAFETY NETTING:

- Advise immediate consultation if diarrhoea worsens, significant weight loss occurs, or if new symptoms like vomiting or severe abdominal pain develop.
- Encourage returning to the clinic with any challenges or uncertainties about dietary changes.

# CASE 7

# HIV: Breaking Bad News

## Doctor's Notes

*Patient Details:*

- **Name:** Ahmed Mansoor
- **Age:** 34
- **Occupation:** Teacher
- **Presenting Complaint:** Recurrent chest infections and follow-up on recent lab and imaging results
- Treated for chlamydia, gonorrhoea, syphilis, and genital herpes in the last 8 months
- **Setting:** Family Medicine Clinic

## PATIENT'S SIMULATED SCRIPT:

### Opening Statement:

"Doctor, I'm still feeling unwell, and this infection just isn't going away. I'm here to find out what the results show."

## HISTORY:

- **Presenting Symptoms:**
  - Persistent cough for 3 weeks, producing yellowish sputum.
  - Shortness of breath on exertion and occasional chest discomfort.
  - Fever and night sweats over the past 2 weeks.
  - Significant weight loss (approximately 6 kg over 3 months).
  - Recurrent similar chest infections over the last year, requiring antibiotics.
- **Lifestyle and Risk Factors:**
  - Non-smoker, occasional alcohol use.
  - History of multiple unprotected sexual encounters over the past 2 years.

## DRUG HISTORY:

- **Regular Medications:** None.
- **Allergies:** None known.
- **Recent Medications:** Completed a course of antibiotics prescribed for previous infections.

## FAMILY HISTORY:

- No history of chronic respiratory or immunological conditions.
- Father has hypertension, mother has type 2 diabetes.

## IDEAS, CONCERNS, EXPECTATIONS:

- **Ideas:** Suspects he might have a serious lung condition or a weak immune system.
- **Concerns:** Worried about long-term damage to his lungs and inability to recover fully.
- **Expectations:** Hopes to get an explanation for his recurrent infections and a clear plan for treatment.

## ON EXAMINATION:

- **General Appearance:** Appears thin and fatigued.
- **Vitals:** BP 110/68 mmHg, HR 92 bpm, temperature 38.2°C, $SpO_2$ 92% on room air.
- **Chest Examination:**
  - Reduced air entry in the right lower lung field.
  - Crackles and dullness to percussion in the same area.
  - No wheezing.

## INVESTIGATIONS AND RESULTS:

1. **HIV Testing:** Positive, confirmed via ELISA and Western blot.
2. **Chest X-Ray:** Shows features consistent with *Pneumocystis jirovecii* pneumonia (bilateral interstitial infiltrates).

## WHAT IS THE DIAGNOSIS?

- **Human Immunodeficiency Virus (HIV) Infection** (newly diagnosed).
- ***Pneumocystis Jirovecii* Pneumonia (PCP)** as a manifestation of advanced HIV.

HIV is a virus that attacks the body's immune system, specifically the white blood cells that help fight infections. If left untreated, HIV can weaken the immune system over time, making it harder for the body to fight off diseases. This can lead to acquired immunodeficiency syndrome (AIDS), the most severe stage of HIV, where the body becomes extremely vulnerable to infections and certain cancers. There is no cure, but with proper treatment (antiretroviral therapy [ART]), people with HIV can live long, healthy lives and reduce the risk of spreading the virus.

## HOW WOULD YOU MANAGE THIS PATIENT?

1. **Immediate Treatment:**
   - Admit to hospital for initiation of treatment.
   - Start trimethoprim-sulfamethoxazole (TMP-SMX) for PCP.
   - Provide supplemental oxygen therapy as needed.

2. **HIV Management:**
   - Urgently refer to an infectious disease specialist for comprehensive HIV care.
   - Initiate ART after PCP treatment stabilizes.
   - Perform baseline investigations, including CD4 count, viral load, and resistance testing.
3. **Supportive Measures:**
   - Offer psychological support and counselling regarding the new diagnosis.
   - Discuss transmission risks and prevention strategies.
4. **Preventive Care:**
   - Screen for other opportunistic infections (e.g., tuberculosis, hepatitis B/C).
   - Provide vaccinations as appropriate (e.g., pneumococcal, influenza).

**What communication principles should be followed when breaking bad news to this patient?**

Use the SPIKES protocol: Set up the interview, assess Perception, obtain Invitation, give Knowledge, address Emotions, and offer Strategy/Summary with empathy and clarity.

**Why is it important to delay initiation of ART until after stabilization of PCP?**

Starting ART too early during acute PCP may lead to immune reconstitution inflammatory syndrome (IRIS); stabilization first reduces this risk.

**What are the immediate priorities in managing a newly diagnosed HIV patient with opportunistic infection?**

Start treatment for PCP, provide supportive care, refer to HIV specialist, perform CD4/viral load testing, and initiate counselling and contact tracing.

## FOLLOW-UP:

- Arrange for close monitoring during hospitalization and subsequent outpatient follow-up.
- Coordinate care with a multidisciplinary team, including an infectious disease specialist and counsellor.

## SAFETY NETTING:

- Advise seeking immediate medical attention if symptoms worsen, such as increasing shortness of breath or chest pain.
- Encourage open communication about any new symptoms or challenges related to diagnosis or treatment.

# CASE 8 Hypertension

## Doctor's Notes

*Patient Details:*

- **Name:** Khalid Ahmed
- **Age:** 36
- **Occupation:** Software Engineer
- **Presenting Complaint:** Poorly controlled hypertension despite being on three antihypertensive medications
- **Setting:** Family Medicine Clinic

## PATIENT'S SIMULATED SCRIPT:

### Opening Statement:

"Doctor, my blood pressure is still not under control even though I'm taking all these medications. What did the tests show?"

## HISTORY:

- **Presenting Symptoms:**
  - Consistently high blood pressure readings despite adherence to prescribed medications.
  - Occasional headaches and fatigue.
  - No chest pain, palpitations, or shortness of breath.
  - No history of fainting or dizziness.
- **Lifestyle and Risk Factors:**
  - Sedentary lifestyle due to long working hours.
  - Eats out frequently; diet high in salt and fat.
  - Non-smoker, occasional alcohol use.
  - Family history of hypertension (father) and type 2 diabetes (mother).

## DRUG HISTORY:

- **Regular Medications:**
  - Amlodipine 10 mg daily.
  - Losartan 100 mg daily.
  - Hydrochlorothiazide 25 mg daily.
- **Allergies:** None known.
- **Compliance:** Reports good adherence to medication schedule.

## FAMILY HISTORY:

- Father has hypertension.
- Mother has type 2 diabetes.
- No family history of renal disease.

## IDEAS, CONCERNS, EXPECTATIONS:

- **Ideas:** Wonders if the medications are not working or if there is an underlying issue.
- **Concerns:** Worried about long-term complications such as kidney damage or heart disease.
- **Expectations:** Hopes for a better explanation of his condition and a more effective treatment plan.

## ON EXAMINATION:

- **General Appearance:** Appears well but mildly anxious.
- **Vitals:** BP 158/96 mmHg, HR 78 bpm, BMI 29 (overweight).
  - **Cardiovascular Examination:**
  - Normal heart sounds.
  - No murmurs or bruits.
- **Abdominal Examination:**
  - No palpable masses or tenderness.
  - No audible renal bruits.

## INVESTIGATIONS AND RESULTS:

1. **Renal Ultrasound with Doppler:** Revealed significant right renal artery stenosis.
2. **Blood Tests:**
   - **HbA1c:** 6.2% (pre-diabetes range)
   - **Total Cholesterol:** 6.5 mmol/L (elevated)
   - **LDL:** 4.2 mmol/L (elevated)
   - **HDL:** 0.9 mmol/L (low)
   - **Triglycerides:** 2.4 mmol/L (elevated)
   - **Renal Function:** eGFR: 90 mL/min/1.73m$^2$ (normal renal function)

## WHAT IS THE DIAGNOSIS?

**Secondary Hypertension due to Renal Artery Stenosis** (right-sided).

1. **Pre-Diabetes**
2. **Hyperlipidaemia**

Renal artery stenosis is a condition where the arteries that supply blood to the kidneys become narrowed. This reduces blood flow to the kidneys, which can cause high blood pressure (hypertension) and kidney damage. The most common causes are a buildup of fatty deposits (atherosclerosis) or a condition called fibromuscular dysplasia, which affects the artery walls. Symptoms may not always be noticeable, but severe cases can lead to uncontrolled high blood pressure, kidney failure, or fluid buildup in the body. Treatment includes medications to control blood pressure, lifestyle changes, and in some cases, procedures like angioplasty to open the narrowed artery.

## HOW WOULD YOU MANAGE THIS PATIENT?

1. **Immediate Management:**
   - Refer to a nephrologist or vascular specialist for further evaluation and potential intervention (e.g., angioplasty or stenting of the renal artery).
   - Consider adding or adjusting antihypertensive therapy in consultation with a specialist.
2. **Lifestyle Modifications:**
   - Counsel on a low-salt, DASH diet to help lower blood pressure.
   - Emphasize regular physical activity (e.g., 30 minutes of moderate exercise most days of the week).
   - Advise weight loss to achieve a healthy BMI.
3. **Management of Pre-Diabetes:**
   - Recommend lifestyle interventions, including dietary changes and increased physical activity.
   - Discuss monitoring glucose levels and follow-up HbA1c in 3–6 months.
4. **Hyperlipidaemia Management:**
   - Initiate a high-intensity statin (e.g., atorvastatin 40–80 mg daily).
   - Counsel on dietary changes to lower cholesterol (reduce saturated fats, increase fibre).
5. **Monitoring and Follow-up:**
   - Regular BP monitoring at home and in the clinic.
   - Review response to lifestyle changes and medication adjustments in 4–6 weeks.

**What features in this case suggest secondary hypertension rather than primary (essential) hypertension?**

Young age (<40), resistant hypertension on three drugs, and evidence of renal artery stenosis on Doppler imaging.

**Why is renal artery stenosis a significant cause of secondary hypertension, and how is it managed?**

It reduces renal perfusion, triggering RAAS activation and elevated BP. Management includes BP control, lifestyle changes, and possible angioplasty or stenting.

**What cardiovascular risk factors require intervention in this patient beyond hypertension?**

Pre-diabetes (HbA1c 6.2%), hyperlipidaemia (elevated LDL and triglycerides, low HDL), and overweight (BMI 29). All require lifestyle changes and statin therapy.

## SAFETY NETTING:

- Advise seeking urgent medical attention if symptoms such as severe headache, chest pain, or sudden weakness occur.
- Encourage reporting any side effects from medications.
- Discuss signs of worsening kidney function, such as reduced urine output or swelling.

# CASE 9 Hyperthyroidism

## Doctor's Notes

*Patient Details:*

- **Name:** Layla Hassan
- **Age:** 28
- **Occupation:** Marketing Specialist
- **Presenting Complaint:** Weight loss and shaking
- **Setting:** Family Medicine Clinic

## PATIENT'S SIMULATED SCRIPT:

### Opening Statement:

"Doctor, I've been losing weight even though I'm eating normally, and my hands won't stop shaking. What did the test results show?"

## HISTORY:

- **Presenting Symptoms:**
  - Unintentional weight loss (approximately 6 kg in 2 months).
  - Fine tremors in the hands.
  - Palpitations and occasional feeling of a racing heart.
  - Increased appetite but no changes in diet.
  - Heat intolerance and excessive sweating.
  - Fatigue and irritability.
  - Irregular menstrual periods over the past few months.
- **Lifestyle and Risk Factors:**
  - Non-smoker, does not consume alcohol.
  - Balanced diet, no recent significant changes in lifestyle.
  - No recent travel or infections.

## DRUG HISTORY:

- **Regular Medications:** None.
- **Allergies:** None known.
- **Compliance:** Not applicable.

## FAMILY HISTORY:

- Mother has type 2 diabetes.
- Sister has hypothyroidism.

## IDEAS, CONCERNS, EXPECTATIONS:

- **Ideas:** Wonders if the symptoms could be related to having a very high metabolism.
- **Concerns:** Afraid that her symptoms might worsen or indicate a serious condition.
- **Expectations:** Hopes to understand the results of the tests and receive a treatment plan to feel better.

## ON EXAMINATION:

- **General Appearance:** Appears anxious, slightly flushed.
- **Vitals:** BP 128/76 mmHg, HR 102 bpm (regular), temperature 36.8°C, BMI 20 (normal range).
- **Thyroid Examination:**
    - Visible thyroid enlargement (goitre).
    - No palpable nodules.
    - No tenderness.
- **Neurological Examination:**
    - Fine tremors in both hands.
    - Reflexes brisk bilaterally.

## INVESTIGATIONS AND RESULTS:

1. **Thyroid Function Tests:**
    - **TSH:** Suppressed (<0.01 mIU/L).
    - **Free T4:** Elevated (25 pmol/L, normal range 9–19 pmol/L).
    - **Free T3:** Elevated (8.2 pmol/L, normal range 3.1–6.8 pmol/L).
2. **Thyroid Ultrasound:**
    - Diffuse thyroid enlargement with increased vascularity (findings consistent with Graves' disease).
3. **Thyroid Antibodies:**
    - Positive for TSH receptor antibodies (TRAb).

## WHAT IS THE DIAGNOSIS?

**Primary Hyperthyroidism** secondary to **Graves' Disease.**

Graves' disease is an autoimmune condition that causes hyperthyroidism, which means the thyroid gland produces too much thyroid hormone. This speeds up the body's metabolism, leading to symptoms like weight loss, rapid heartbeat, sweating, anxiety, and shaky hands. It happens because the immune system mistakenly attacks the thyroid, making it overactive. Some people with Graves' disease also develop eye problems (Graves' ophthalmopathy), causing bulging eyes, irritation, or vision issues.

## HOW WOULD YOU MANAGE THIS PATIENT?

1. **Initial Management:**
   - Prescribe antithyroid medication (e.g., carbimazole 15–20 mg daily) to reduce thyroid hormone production.
   - Consider beta-blockers (e.g., propranolol 20–40 mg three times daily) for symptomatic relief of tremors and palpitations.
2. **Lifestyle Advice:**
   - Avoid excessive iodine intake, such as from iodized salt, seaweed, kelp-based supplements, and certain seafood (e.g., shrimp, cod, and tuna).
   - Discuss the importance of stress management to minimize symptom exacerbation.
3. **Specialist Referral:**
   - Refer to an endocrinologist for further evaluation and ongoing management.
   - Discuss potential future treatment options, such as radioactive iodine therapy or surgery, if appropriate.
4. **Monitoring:**
   - Regular follow-up for thyroid function tests to adjust treatment accordingly.
   - Monitor for side effects of medications, including agranulocytosis (educate on symptoms such as sore throat or fever).

**What clinical and investigation findings support the diagnosis of Graves' disease in this patient?**

Symptoms (weight loss, tremor, palpitations), diffuse goitre, suppressed TSH, elevated T3/T4, positive TRAb, and increased vascularity on thyroid ultrasound.

**What are the roles of carbimazole and propranolol in the initial management?**

Carbimazole reduces thyroid hormone synthesis; propranolol controls symptoms like tremor, palpitations, and anxiety.

**What complications should patients on carbimazole be educated about, and what warning signs should they report?**

Agranulocytosis is a rare but serious side effect – patients should report sore throat, fever, or mouth ulcers immediately.

# CASE 10 Poorly Controlled Diabetic

## Doctor's Notes

*Patient Details:*

- **Name:** Omar Al-Hassan
- **Age:** 52
- **Occupation:** Accountant
- **Presenting Complaint:** Blurred vision, polyuria, and polydipsia
- **Setting:** Family Medicine Clinic

## PATIENT'S SIMULATED SCRIPT:

### Opening Statement:

"Doctor, I'm here for my blood test results. I've also been noticing some changes recently."

## HISTORY:

- **Presenting Symptoms:**
  - Blurred vision for the past 3 weeks, which worsens intermittently, especially after meals.
  - Increased thirst (polydipsia) and frequent urination (polyuria) over the past month.
  - Occasional dry mouth and fatigue.
  - No headaches, dizziness, or eye pain.
  - Weight gain, around 5 kg in the last 2 months.
- **Additional Information:**
  - The blood tests were ordered to assess his diabetes control after he mentioned at the last visit that he was feeling unwell and suspected worsening blood sugar levels.
- **Lifestyle and Risk Factors:**
  - Known to have type 2 diabetes for 12 years.
  - Diet is inconsistent; occasionally indulges in high-sugar and high-fat foods.
  - Sedentary lifestyle due to long hours at work.
  - Non-smoker, occasional alcohol use.

## DRUG HISTORY:

- **Regular Medications:**
  - Metformin 1000 mg twice daily.
  - Gliclazide 80 mg twice daily.
  - Atorvastatin 20 mg once daily.
  - Ramipril 5 mg once daily.
- **Allergies:** None known.
- **Compliance:** Admits to occasionally missing doses of medications due to a busy schedule.

## FAMILY HISTORY:

- Mother had type 2 diabetes and hypertension.
- Father passed away from a myocardial infarction at 62 years old.

## IDEAS, CONCERNS, EXPECTATIONS:

- **Ideas:** Believes his symptoms are related to becoming older, he's heard everything tends to go wrong when you're older.
- **Concerns:** Worried that without prompt medical help he'll get progressively worse.
- **Expectations:** Hopes you can confirm what is wrong with him and help him feel better.

## ON EXAMINATION:

- **General Appearance:** Overweight (BMI 29), appears tired.
- **Vitals:** BP 140/85 mmHg, HR 78 bpm (regular), temperature 36.9°C.

**The resident is expected to perform a comprehensive ophthalmological examination, including assessment of visual fields, to successfully pass the station.**

- **Eye Examination:**
  - No redness or discharge.
  - Fundoscopy shows mild background diabetic retinopathy.
- **Cardiovascular and Respiratory:** Normal heart sounds, clear lungs.
- **Abdomen:** Soft, non-tender, no organomegaly.

## INVESTIGATIONS AND RESULTS:

1. **Blood Tests:**
   - **HbA1c:** 10.2% (poor control).
   - **Fasting Blood Glucose:** 14.5 mmol/L (high).
   - **Lipid Profile:** Elevated LDL (3.8 mmol/L), triglycerides elevated (2.5 mmol/L).
   - **Renal Function:** eGFR 70 mL/min/1.73m$^2$ (normal), microalbuminuria detected.
2. **Urinalysis:**
   - Positive for glucose, no ketones.
3. **Retinal Screening:**
   - Shows mild background diabetic retinopathy.

## WHAT IS THE DIAGNOSIS?

1. **Poorly Controlled Type 2 Diabetes Mellitus** with complications:
   - Background diabetic retinopathy.
   - Hyperglycaemia causing blurred vision.

2. **Dyslipidaemia.**

Poorly controlled diabetes occurs when blood sugar levels stay too high for a long time due to inadequate management with diet, exercise, or medication. This can lead to serious health problems, including nerve damage (neuropathy), kidney disease, vision loss, and an increased risk of heart attack and stroke. Symptoms may include frequent urination, extreme thirst, fatigue, blurry vision, and slow-healing wounds. Proper management through lifestyle changes, medications, and regular monitoring of blood sugar can help prevent complications.

## HOW WOULD YOU MANAGE THIS PATIENT?

1. **Acute Management:**
   - Intensify blood sugar control by adding a glucagon-like peptide-1 (GLP-1) receptor agonist (e.g., liraglutide) or initiating insulin therapy temporarily.
   - Adjust current oral hypoglycaemic medications as appropriate (e.g., increase gliclazide dose or consider switching to an SGLT2 inhibitor).
   - Referral to ophthalmologist.
2. **Lifestyle Modifications:**
   - Recommend a diabetes-specific diet with the help of a dietitian.
   - Encourage regular physical activity (e.g., 30 minutes of moderate exercise 5 days per week).
   - Stress the importance of strict medication adherence.
3. **Monitoring and Follow-up:**
   - Arrange for repeat HbA1c and renal function tests in 3 months.
   - Refer to ophthalmology for further assessment and management of diabetic retinopathy.
   - Regular follow-up for lipid management and blood pressure control.
4. **Preventive Measures:**
   - Reinforce foot care and annual diabetic foot screening.
   - Ensure up-to-date vaccinations (e.g., influenza, pneumococcal).

**What are the key clinical features in this case that indicate poorly controlled diabetes?**

HbA1C 10.2% and polyuria, blurred vision, fatigue, weight gain, and microalbuminuria.

**Which complications of diabetes are evident in this patient, and how are they detected?**

- **Microvascular:**
  - **Retinopathy** – detected on fundoscopy.
  - **Nephropathy** – evidenced by microalbuminuria.
- **Macrovascular risk factors:** Dyslipidaemia (elevated LDL and triglycerides), hypertension (BP 140/85 mmHg) – increase risk of cardiovascular events.

## FOLLOW-UP:

**What follow-up and preventive measures should be arranged for this patient?**

- Repeat HbA1c and renal function in 3 months.
- Regular ophthalmology follow-up for diabetic retinopathy.
- Monitor lipid profile and blood pressure.
- Reinforce foot care and annual screening.
- Ensure vaccinations are up to date (influenza, pneumococcal).

**Given his current regimen (metformin + gliclazide), discuss the next step in medication adjustment. Include rationale for your choices.**

**Options:**

- Add a GLP-1 receptor agonist (beneficial for glycaemic control and weight loss).
- Consider SGLT2 inhibitor (benefits glycaemic control, cardiovascular risk, and renal protection).
- If inadequate, short-term insulin therapy may be necessary.

**Rationale:** Current dual oral therapy is insufficient (HbA1c 10.2%). Intensification targets better glycaemic control and prevention of complications.

# CASE 11

# Pre-Conception Advice

## Doctor's Notes

*Patient Details:*

- **Name:** Amina Khalid
- **Age:** 27
- **Occupation:** Graphic Designer
- **Presenting Complaint:** Pre-conception advice
- **Setting:** Family Medicine Clinic

## PATIENT'S SIMULATED SCRIPT:

### Opening Statement:

"Doctor, I'm planning to start a family soon, and I'd like to know how I can prepare for a healthy pregnancy."

## HISTORY:

- **Reason for Visit:**
  - Seeking advice on how to optimize health before conceiving.
- **Lifestyle and Risk Factors:**
  - Non-smoker, does not consume alcohol.
  - Regularly exercises (yoga and light cardio).
  - Balanced diet, but occasionally skips meals due to a busy schedule.
  - No recent travel or infections.
- **Gynaecological History:**
  - Regular menstrual cycles, no known issues with fertility.
  - No history of sexually transmitted infections.
- **Past Medical History:**
  - Diagnosed with epilepsy at age 20, currently well-controlled.

## DRUG HISTORY:

- **Regular Medications:** Sodium valproate 500 mg twice daily.
- **Allergies:** None known.
- **Compliance:** Fully adherent to medication regimen.

## FAMILY HISTORY:

- Mother has type 2 diabetes.
- No family history of epilepsy or other significant medical conditions.

## IDEAS, CONCERNS, EXPECTATIONS:

- **Ideas:** Wants to ensure her health and medication regimen are suitable for pregnancy.
- **Concerns:** Worried about how epilepsy and current medication might affect pregnancy and the baby.
- **Expectations:** Expects a clear plan to prepare for pregnancy and manage her epilepsy safely.

## ON EXAMINATION:

- **General Appearance:** Healthy and well-nourished.
- **Vitals:** BP 118/76 mmHg, HR 72 bpm (regular), BMI 22 (normal range).
- **Neurological Examination:** Normal, no focal deficits.
- **Abdominal Examination:** Normal.

## INVESTIGATIONS AND RESULTS:

1. **Routine Preconception Blood Tests:**
   - **Full Blood Count:** Normal.
   - **Serum Folate:** Normal.
   - **Renal and Liver Function Tests:** Normal.
   - **Thyroid Function Tests:** Normal.
2. **Epilepsy Monitoring:**
   - No recent seizures or side effects from medication.

## WHAT IS THE DIAGNOSIS?

**Epilepsy** – well-controlled on sodium valproate.

## HOW WOULD YOU MANAGE THIS PATIENT?

1. **Medication Review:**
   - Transition from sodium valproate to a safer alternative for pregnancy, such as lamotrigine, under close supervision.
   - Gradual dose adjustment to maintain seizure control while minimizing risks to the foetus.
   - Educate the patient about the risks of sodium valproate in pregnancy, including teratogenicity and developmental issues.
2. **Lifestyle and Health Optimization:**
   - Maintain a balanced diet rich in essential nutrients.
   - Encourage continued regular exercise appropriate for preconception health.
   - Avoid exposure to infections and ensure up-to-date vaccinations (e.g., rubella, varicella).

3. **Specialist Referral:**
   - Refer to a neurologist for ongoing management of epilepsy during pregnancy.
   - Coordinate with obstetrics for high-risk pregnancy care.
4. **Monitoring and Follow-up:**
   - Regular monitoring of seizure control and medication levels.
   - Routine antenatal care once pregnant, including screening for foetal anomalies.

**What are the main risks associated with sodium valproate in women planning pregnancy?**

Highly teratogenic; risks include neural tube defects (e.g., spina bifida), congenital malformations (cardiac, craniofacial), and developmental/behavioral problems in the child. It is generally avoided in women planning pregnancy.

**What preconception interventions should be recommended to the patient besides medication adjustment?**

- High-dose folic acid (5 mg daily) at least 3 months before conception.
- Avoid teratogenic exposures (e.g., alcohol, smoking).
- Ensure up-to-date vaccinations (rubella, varicella).

**How should seizure control be managed during the transition from valproate to a safer alternative?**

Taper valproate while titrating the alternative medication. Monitor for breakthrough seizures whilst adjusting doses to maintain optimal seizure control.

# CASE 12 Prostatitis

## Doctor's Notes

*Patient Details:*

- **Name:** Ahmed Al-Mansoor
- **Age:** 45
- **Occupation:** Office Manager
- **Presenting Complaint:** Dysuria not improving on antibiotics
- **Setting:** Family Medicine Clinic

## PATIENT'S SIMULATED SCRIPT:

### Opening Statement:

"Doctor, I've been having pain and burning when I urinate for the past 2 weeks; it's really frustrating me now, I hope you can help!"

## HISTORY:

### Reason for Visit:

Mr. Ahmed is seeking advice on why his symptoms of dysuria, which started 2 weeks ago, are not improving despite being prescribed antibiotics (ciprofloxacin) for what was initially thought to be a urinary tract infection (UTI).

### Lifestyle and Risk Factors:

- Non-smoker.
- Occasionally drinks alcohol (one to two drinks on weekends).
- Works in an office setting with limited physical activity.
- No recent travel or exposure to infections.
- Enjoys baklava and eating fast food.

### Past Medical History:

- No known history of diabetes, hypertension, or kidney disease.
- No previous UTIs or prostate issues.

### Drug History:

- **Ciprofloxacin** 500 mg twice daily (prescribed for presumed UTI) 2 weeks ago.
- **Allergies:** None known.
- **Compliance:** Fully adherent to medication regimen.

### Family History:

- Father has type 2 diabetes.
- No family history of prostate disease or urinary tract cancer.

## IDEAS, CONCERNS, EXPECTATIONS:

### Ideas:

- Mr. Ahmed believes his infection might be resistant to the antibiotics, as his symptoms are not improving.

### Concerns:

- He is concerned that he might have a more complicated infection as his issues remain unresolved.
- He is worried that his health could be compromised in some way, given the persistence of symptoms.

### Expectations:

- He expects an explanation as to why the antibiotics haven't worked and is hoping for a treatment plan that effectively addresses his symptoms and prevents future infections.

## ON EXAMINATION:

- **General Appearance:** Healthy, no signs of acute distress
  - **Vitals:** BP 132/85 mmHg, HR 88 bpm, temperature 36.8°C.
  - Blood Glucose: 148 mg/dL (found during routine checks, as part of further investigations).
- **Abdomen:** Soft, non-tender with no palpable masses
- **Genitourinary:**
  - No external genital abnormalities.
  - Tenderness over the suprapubic area and perineum.
  - Digital rectal examination (DRE): Mildly enlarged and tender prostate.
- **Neurological:** No focal deficits

## INVESTIGATIONS AND RESULTS:

- **Urinalysis:** Positive for leukocytes, nitrites, and *E. coli.*
- **Urine Culture:** *E. coli* (sensitive to ciprofloxacin)
- **Blood Tests:**
  - **Full Blood Count:** Normal
  - **Renal Function:** Normal
  - **Liver Function:** Normal
  - **HbA1c:** 7% Diabetic

## WHAT IS THE DIAGNOSIS?

- **Bacterial Prostatitis** (likely due to *E. coli*).
- **New Diagnosis of Type 2 Diabetes Mellitus** based on blood glucose findings.

Bacterial prostatitis is an infection of the prostate gland caused by bacteria. It can be acute (sudden and severe) or chronic (long-lasting with milder symptoms). Common symptoms include pain in the pelvic area, difficulty urinating, frequent urination, fever, chills, and sometimes painful ejaculation. It is usually caused by bacteria from the urinary tract, such as *E. coli*. Diagnosis is made through urine tests, blood tests, and sometimes prostate fluid analysis. Treatment involves antibiotics, with longer courses needed for chronic cases. In severe cases, hospitalization may be required for IV antibiotics.

## HOW WOULD YOU MANAGE THIS PATIENT?

1. **Antibiotic Therapy:**
   - Since the urine culture shows *E. coli* is susceptible to ciprofloxacin, the current antibiotic can be continued. However, to ensure adequate treatment, consider extending the course to **4–6 weeks** due to the chronic nature of prostatitis.
   - Alternatively, switch to **trimethoprim–sulfamethoxazole** or another agent based on patient preference and tolerance.
2. What features would suggest the diagnosis of bacterial prostatitis rather than a simple urinary tract infection?
   - Persistent dysuria, despite a full course of antibiotics.
   - Tenderness in the suprapubic and perineal region.
   - Tender prostate on digital rectal examination.
   - *E. coli*–positive urine culture.
3. Why is a prolonged course of antibiotics recommended for this patient, and what duration is appropriate?

   Chronic bacterial prostatitis requires prolonged courses of antibiotics (4–6 weeks) to resolve deep-lying infection in the prostate tissue.
4. What are the common complications if bacterial prostatitis is inadequately treated?
   - Recurrent infections.
   - Prostatic abscess.
   - Pelvic pain syndrome.
   - Urinary obstruction/retention.
   - Sepsis.
5. **Diabetes Management:**
   - Mr. Ahmed will need to address his **newly diagnosed diabetes**. Recommend starting **metformin** 500 mg twice daily and providing lifestyle modifications (diet, exercise) to manage glucose levels effectively.
   - Encourage **weight loss**, **regular exercise**, and **dietary modifications** (low glycaemic foods, balanced meals) to improve glucose control.
6. **Lifestyle Modifications:**
   - Increase fluid intake to help flush the urinary system.
   - Implement a **healthy diet** to manage both prostatitis and new diabetes diagnosis.
   - Regular exercise is recommended to manage both diabetes and overall health.

## FOLLOW-UP:

- Follow up in **2–3 weeks** to assess symptom resolution and glucose control.
- If symptoms persist, consider referral to a urologist or further imaging (e.g., ultrasound) for prostatitis evaluation.

# CASE 13
# Angina

## Doctor's Notes

*Patient Details:*

- **Name:** Omar Khaled
- **Age:** 58
- **Occupation:** Retired engineer
- **Presenting Complaint:** Chest pain with exertion
- **Setting:** Family Medicine Clinic

## PATIENT'S SIMULATED SCRIPT:

### Opening Statement:

"Doctor, I've been having some chest pain when I'm walking or doing any kind of physical activity. It usually goes away after a few minutes of resting, but it's been happening more frequently lately, and I'm getting a little worried."

## HISTORY:

### Reason for Visit:

Mr. Omar is concerned about recurrent chest pain that occurs with physical exertion and resolves with rest.

### Lifestyle and Risk Factors:

- Smoker, 1 pack per day for 30 years, currently trying to quit.
- Occasionally drinks alcohol (2–3 drinks per week).
- Not very physically active, mostly sedentary lifestyle.
- Overweight, BMI of 29.5 kg/m$^2$.
- No recent travel or history of chest trauma.

### Cardiac History:

- No previous history of myocardial infarction or arrhythmias.
- No known history of heart disease, but family history of coronary artery disease (father had a heart attack at age 60).

### Past Medical History:

- Hypertension, diagnosed 10 years ago, poorly controlled with occasional compliance issues with medications.
- Mild osteoarthritis in knees.

### Drug History:

- **Amlodipine** 5 mg daily for hypertension.
- **Ibuprofen** 400 mg as needed for knee pain.
- **Allergies:** None known
- **Compliance:** Irregular with blood pressure medications.

### Family History:

- Father had a myocardial infarction at age 60 and passed away at age 62.
- Mother had hypertension and diabetes.

## IDEAS, CONCERNS, EXPECTATIONS:

- **Ideas:** Mr. Omar believes his chest pain might be due to muscle strain or acid reflux.
- **Concerns:**
  - He is concerned that his chest pain might be related to heart disease, especially since it has been occurring more frequently and radiates to his left hand.
  - He is also worried about the impact of his hypertension and family history of heart disease.
- **Expectations:** Mr. Omar expects a clear explanation of his symptoms and a treatment plan to either confirm or rule out a heart condition.

## ON EXAMINATION:

- **General Appearance:** Overweight, no signs of acute distress.
- **Vitals:** BP 145/90 mmHg, HR 84 bpm (regular), temperature 36.6°C, oxygen saturation 98% on room air.
- **Cardiovascular Exam:**
  - No jugular venous distention.
  - Normal heart sounds, no murmurs or gallops.
  - Regular rhythm.
  - Peripheral pulses palpable and equal in both arms and legs.
- **Respiratory Exam:** Clear lung fields, no wheezing or crackles.
- **Abdomen:** Soft, non-tender, no palpable masses.
- **Musculoskeletal Exam:** No joint tenderness or deformities in knees.

## INVESTIGATIONS AND RESULTS:

- **ECG:** Normal sinus rhythm, no acute ischemic changes (ST depression or T wave inversion).
- **Blood Tests:**
  - **Full Blood Count:** Normal.
  - **Lipid Profile:** Total cholesterol 220 mg/dL, LDL 140 mg/dL, HDL 40 mg/dL, triglycerides 170 mg/dL (borderline high).
  - **Blood Glucose:** 105 mg/dL (fasting, mildly elevated).
  - **Renal Function:** Normal.
- **Stress Test:** Recommended for further evaluation of exertional chest pain, results pending.

### Stress Test Protocol:

- **Type of Test:** Treadmill exercise stress test (Bruce Protocol)
- **Duration:** 8 minutes
- **Max HR Achieved:** 140 bpm (87% of predicted maximum)
- **BP Response:** Resting 130/80 mmHg → Peak 170/90 mmHg
- **Exercise Termination:** Due to chest discomfort and ST changes

### ECG Findings:

- **Resting ECG:** Normal sinus rhythm, no ST-T wave abnormalities
- **During Exercise:**
  - 2.5 mm **ST depression in leads II, III, aVF, and V4-V6** (horizontal/downsloping)
  - **Onset at 6 METs** of exertion, worsening with increased workload
  - No ventricular arrhythmias
- **Post-Exercise (Recovery) Phase:**
  - ST depressions persist for >**5 minutes**, suggestive of significant ischemia
  - Slow heart rate recovery (**HR drop <12 bpm at 1 min post exercise**), indicating poor cardiovascular fitness

### Symptoms During Test:

- **Exertional Chest Pain:** Reported at 6 minutes, rated **5/10**, relieved after stopping exercise.
- **Dyspnoea and Fatigue:** Moderate at peak exertion.
- **Syncope or Severe Arrhythmia:** None observed.

## WHAT IS THE DIAGNOSIS?

- **Stable Angina** likely due to **Coronary Artery Disease (CAD)**, given the pattern of exertional chest pain that radiates to the left arm, a classic symptom of angina.
- **Hypertension** (poorly controlled), which is a significant risk factor for CAD.
- **Borderline Dyslipidaemia** (elevated total cholesterol and LDL).
- **Mild Hyperglycaemia** (suggesting potential prediabetes).

Stable angina is a type of chest pain that occurs when the heart does not get enough oxygen-rich blood. It usually occurs during physical activity or stress and goes away with rest or medication (such as nitroglycerin). The pain or discomfort may feel like pressure, tightness, or a squeezing sensation in the chest and can sometimes spread to the arms, neck, jaw, or back. It is caused by narrowed heart arteries (coronary artery disease) due to a buildup of fatty deposits. While stable angina itself is not a heart attack, it is a warning sign of heart disease and should be managed with lifestyle changes, medications, or sometimes procedures like stents.

**What clinical features and investigation findings support the diagnosis of stable angina in Mr. Omar?**

- **Symptoms:** Exertional chest pain radiating to the left arm subsequently relieved by rest.
- **Risk Factors:** Hypertension, smoking, obesity, dyslipidaemia, family history of CAD.
- **Stress Test:** ST depression in multiple leads during exertion.

**What is the significance of the stress test findings (exercise-induced ST depression and slow heart rate recovery)?**

- ST depression indicates myocardial ischaemia due to coronary artery obstruction.
- >5 min duration suggests significant ischaemia.
- Slow heart rate recovery <12 bpm drop at 1 min reflects poor cardiovascular fitness and increased risk of heart attack and stroke in particular.

**Outline the immediate pharmacological management for this patient.**

- **Anti-Ischemic Therapy:** Beta-blocker (metoprolol), nitrates (sublingual nitroglycerin for acute relief; consider long-acting if symptoms persist).

- **Antiplatelet:** Aspirin 81 mg daily.
- **Statin:** High-intensity statin (atorvastatin 40–80 mg).
- **Blood Pressure Control:** Optimize antihypertensives (increase amlodipine and/or add ACE inhibitor/ARB).

### What lifestyle modifications are essential for reducing Mr. Omar's cardiovascular risk?

- **Smoking Cessation:** Nicotine replacement therapy and counselling.
- **Diet:** Low-salt, low-fat, high-fibre diet; reduce cholesterol and saturated fats.
- **Exercise:** 30 minutes of moderate activity most days, as tolerated.
- **Weight loss:** Target gradual reduction to BMI <25.

### When should we consider coronary angiography?

- If angina is **not controlled with optimal medical therapy**.
- If stress testing shows **significant ischaemia**, especially multivessel or left main involvement.
- If symptoms worsen or become unstable.

### We should also consider our options for revascularization in the following circumstances:

- **PCI with stenting** for focal disease.
- **CABG** for multivessel disease, left main disease, or diabetics with extensive CAD.

# CASE 14 Dizziness

## Doctor's Notes

*Patient Details:*

- **Name:** Saif Al-Rahman
- **Age:** 45
- **Occupation:** Architect
- **Presenting Complaint:** Dizziness
- **Setting:** Family Medicine Clinic

## PATIENT'S SIMULATED SCRIPT:

### Opening Statement:

"Doctor, I've been feeling dizzy for a few weeks now, and it's starting to affect my daily activities."

## HISTORY:

- **Presenting Symptoms:**
  - Persistent dizziness for the past 3 weeks.
  - Describes the dizziness as a spinning sensation (vertigo), especially when getting up quickly or turning his head.
  - Occasional nausea but no vomiting.
  - Reports ringing in the ears (tinnitus) and mild hearing loss in the right ear.
- **Additional Symptoms:**
  - No headaches, visual changes, or fainting episodes.
  - No numbness, weakness, or difficulty speaking.
- **Triggers:**
  - Symptoms worsen with sudden head movements or changes in position.
  - No clear association with meals, stress, or physical exertion.
- **Lifestyle and Risk Factors:**
  - Non-smoker, occasional alcohol use.
  - Regular coffee drinker (two to three cups per day).
  - No recent travel or infections.

## DRUG HISTORY:

- **Regular Medications:** None.
- **Allergies:** None known.
- **Recent Medications:** Occasionally takes over-the-counter antihistamines for seasonal allergies.

## FAMILY HISTORY:

- Mother has hypertension.
- Father had a stroke at age 68.
- No family history of neurological or balance disorders.

## IDEAS, CONCERNS, EXPECTATIONS:

- **Ideas:** Thinks the dizziness might be due to an infection.
- **Concerns:** Worried it could be something serious affecting his brain.
- **Expectations:** Hopes to find the cause and get effective treatment to stop the dizziness.

## ON EXAMINATION:

- **General Appearance:** Alert and cooperative, appears slightly uncomfortable.
- **Vitals:** BP 124/78 mmHg, HR 80 bpm (regular), temperature 36.7°C.
- **Neurological Examination:**
  - Cranial nerves: Intact.
  - No focal neurological deficits.
  - Normal coordination and gait.
- **Ear Examination:**
  - Right ear: Mild retraction of the tympanic membrane.
  - Left ear: Normal appearance.
- **Rinne's Test:**
  - Right ear: Bone conduction > air conduction (abnormal).
  - Left ear: Air conduction > bone conduction (normal).
- **Weber's Test:**
  - Lateralizes to the right ear.
  - Interpretation: Suggests conductive hearing loss in the right ear.
- **Cardiovascular and Respiratory:** Normal heart sounds, clear lungs.

## INVESTIGATIONS AND RESULTS:

1. **Audiometry:**
   - Confirms mild conductive hearing loss in the right ear.
2. **Blood Tests:**
   - **Fasting Blood Glucose:** Normal.
   - **Full Blood Count:** Normal.
   - **Thyroid Function Tests:** Normal.
3. **Dix–Hallpike Maneuver:**
   - Negative for positional vertigo.

## WHAT IS THE DIAGNOSIS?

**Otitis Media with Effusion** contributing to conductive hearing loss and dizziness.

Otitis media with effusion (OME) is a condition where fluid builds up behind the eardrum without signs of an infection. It often happens after an ear infection or due to poor drainage in the Eustachian tube, which connects the middle ear to the back of the throat. OME can cause dizziness because the fluid affects the balance system in the inner ear, leading to feelings of unsteadiness or lightheadedness. Other symptoms may include muffled hearing, ear fullness, and popping sounds. Most cases resolve on their own, but if persistent, treatment may include decongestants, nasal sprays, or ear tubes to drain the fluid.

## WHAT ARE THE MANAGEMENT OPTIONS FOR OTITIS MEDIA WITH EFFUSION?

1. **Immediate Management:**
   - Prescribe a short course of nasal decongestants or a nasal corticosteroid spray (e.g., mometasone) to reduce any Eustachian tube dysfunction.
   - Consider a referral to an otolaryngologist for further evaluation and management if symptoms persist.
2. **Symptom Management:**
   - Recommend vestibular exercises to help adapt to dizziness.
   - Provide anti-vertigo medication (e.g., betahistine) if symptoms are severely impacting daily activities.
3. **Monitoring:**
   - Arrange for follow-up in 2–4 weeks to reassess symptoms and hearing.
4. **Lifestyle Advice:**
   - Encourage hydration and limiting caffeine to reduce inner ear sensitivity.
   - Avoid sudden head movements that may exacerbate dizziness.
5. Consider referral to ENT if persistent symptoms which may require grommet insertion or further investigation.

### What red flag symptoms would prompt urgent referral?

- Severe or sudden hearing loss.
- Persistent vertigo with neurological signs.
- Infection with systemic features (fever +/– mastoid tenderness).

### What features in the history and examination point towards OME rather than a neurological cause of dizziness?

- Gradual onset of dizziness, not sudden or associated with syncope.
- Presence of tinnitus and hearing loss in the right ear.
- Abnormal Rinne's (BC > AC on right) and Weber's lateralizing to the right (conductive hearing loss).
- Tympanic membrane retraction seen on otoscopy.
- No focal neurological deficits on exam.

### How does OME cause dizziness?

- Fluid accumulation in the middle ear alters middle ear pressure, which affects the transmission of sound and the vestibular system, giving rise to imbalance, unsteadiness, and vertigo.

# CASE 15

# Tonsillitis and Obstructive Sleep Apnoea

## Doctor's Notes

*Patient Details:*

- **Name:** Adam Yusuf
- **Age:** 9
- **Occupation:** Student
- **Presenting Complaint:** Constant tiredness and recurrent throat infections
- **Setting:** Family Medicine Clinic

## PATIENT'S SIMULATED SCRIPT:

### Opening Statement (from parent):

"Doc, Adam is always tired; we can't figure out what the matter is."

## HISTORY:

- **Presenting Symptoms:**
  - Constant tiredness over the past 6 months.
  - Multiple episodes of throat infections this year (around six documented).
  - Difficulty concentrating and decreased school performance compared to previous year.
  - Snoring at night, sometimes gasping for air.
  - Restless sleep and occasional bedwetting, which had previously stopped at age 5.
  - Morning headaches and daytime sleepiness.
  - No weight loss or fever outside of throat infection episodes.
- **Associated Symptoms:**
  - Complains of difficulty swallowing larger pieces of food.
  - No rashes, joint pain, or other systemic symptoms.
- **Past Medical History:**
  - Generally healthy aside from frequent throat infections.
  - No history of hospitalizations or surgeries.

## DRUG HISTORY:

- **Regular Medications:** None.
- **Allergies:** None known.
- **Recent Medications:** Antibiotics prescribed during throat infection episodes.

## FAMILY HISTORY:

- Mother has seasonal allergies.
- Father has a history of obstructive sleep apnoea (OSA).
- No family history of recurrent infections or autoimmune conditions.

## IDEAS, CONCERNS, EXPECTATIONS:

- **Ideas:** Parents suspect the throat infections are causing his tiredness and poor performance.
- **Concerns:** Worried about long-term effects on his health and learning.
- **Expectations:** Expect a solution to improve his energy levels and reduce throat infections.

## ON EXAMINATION:

- **General Appearance:** Tired-looking but alert child.
- **Vitals:** BP 130/85 mmHg (elevated for age), HR 80 bpm (regular), temperature 36.8°C.
- **ENT Examination:**
  - Grade 4 tonsillar hypertrophy, no exudate.
  - Enlarged cervical lymph nodes bilaterally, non-tender.
  - Nasal speech observed.
- **Respiratory Examination:** Clear lung fields, normal breath sounds.
- **Cardiovascular Examination:** Normal heart sounds, no murmurs.
- **Neurological Examination:** Normal.
- **Signs of OSA:**
  - Snoring reported with observed apnoeic episodes during sleep.
  - Morning fatigue and headaches.

## INVESTIGATIONS AND RESULTS:

1. **Full Blood Count:**
   - **Haemoglobin:** 11.2 g/dL (mild anaemia).
   - **White Blood Cells:** Normal.
   - **Platelets:** Normal.
2. **If a sleep study is requested it would confirm** severe OSA with frequent obstructive apnoeas, significant oxygen desaturations, and sleep fragmentation. CPAP therapy is strongly recommended to prevent long-term cardiovascular complications.
3. **Throat Swab Cultures (previous infections):** Showed Group A Streptococcus in two instances.
4. **Blood Pressure Monitoring:** Confirmed elevated BP on multiple occasions.

## WHAT IS THE DIAGNOSIS?

**Obstructive Sleep-Disordered Breathing** secondary to grade 4 tonsillar hypertrophy.

This condition occurs when **severely enlarged tonsils (Grade 4 hypertrophy)** block the airway, making it difficult to breathe during sleep. This leads to **obstructive sleep-disordered breathing (SDB)**, which includes **snoring, gasping,**

**pauses in breathing (apnoea), and restless sleep**. Children and adults with this condition may experience **daytime sleepiness, difficulty concentrating, or behavioural problems** due to poor sleep quality. Treatment often involves **tonsillectomy (surgical removal of the tonsils)** to restore normal airflow and improve sleep.

## OUTLINE THE MANAGEMENT OPTIONS FOR THIS PATIENT:

1. **Referral to ENT Specialist:**
   - Recommend evaluation for possible tonsillectomy, given the recurrent infections, obstructive symptoms, and impact on quality of life.
2. **Symptomatic Management:**
   - Advise continued supportive care during infections (e.g., fluids, analgesics).
   - Monitor anaemia; consider dietary improvements and iron supplementation if needed.
3. **Parental Education:**
   - Discuss the potential benefits and risks of surgical intervention.
   - Explain the possible link between tonsillar hypertrophy, sleep apnoea, and elevated BP.
4. **Lifestyle and Dietary Advice:**
   - Encourage a balanced diet rich in iron (e.g., lean meats, leafy greens, fortified cereals).
   - Ensure good sleep hygiene and minimize distractions before bedtime.

### How should Adam's high blood pressure be addressed in the context of OSA?

**Blood Pressure Management:**

- Monitor BP closely and consider secondary causes related to sleep apnoea.
- Lifestyle interventions, including dietary adjustments and weight management if needed.

### How does tonsillar hypertrophy contribute to OSA in children?

- Enlarged tonsils obstruct the upper airway during sleep.
- Leads to intermittent hypoxia, sleep fragmentation, and poor sleep quality.
- Results in daytime symptoms: Fatigue, behavioural issues, poor concentration, and cardiovascular effects like hypertension.

# CASE 16 Acne

## Doctor's Notes

*Patient Details:*

- **Name:** Layla Hasan
- **Age:** 26
- **Occupation:** Office Worker
- **Presenting Complaint:** Persistent acne
- **Setting:** Family Medicine Clinic

## PATIENT'S SIMULATED SCRIPT:

### Opening Statement:

"I've been struggling with acne for a while, and it's not getting better. I'm worried about how I'll look for my wedding."

## HISTORY:

- **Presenting Symptoms:**
  - Acne primarily on the face, shoulders, and upper back.
  - Worsening over the past year despite over-the-counter treatments.
  - Hirsutism noticed on the face (upper lip and chin) and lower abdomen; she uses cosmetics and waxing to manage it.
  - Oily skin but no scarring from acne.
- **Associated Symptoms:**
  - No amenorrhea; menstrual cycles are regular, every 28–30 days.
  - No significant weight changes or fatigue.
  - No headaches, visual disturbances, or galactorrhoea.
- **Lifestyle Factors:**
  - Balanced diet, moderate physical activity.
  - Stressed about her appearance due to her upcoming wedding in 6 months.
  - No history of smoking, alcohol, or drug use.

## DRUG HISTORY:

- **Regular Medications:** None.
- **Allergies:** None known.
- **Cosmetic Products:** Frequently uses non-prescription acne products and concealers.

## FAMILY HISTORY:

- Mother and elder sister have a history of acne and hirsutism.
- No family history of diabetes or thyroid conditions.

## IDEAS, CONCERNS, EXPECTATIONS:

- **Ideas:** Her skin is bad due to poor genetics.
- **Concerns:** Worried about her appearance and the impact on her self-confidence for her wedding.
- **Expectations:** Wants effective treatment to improve her skin and extra hair on her face before the wedding.

## ON EXAMINATION:

- **General Appearance:** Well-appearing, no acute distress.
- **Skin Examination:**
  - Moderate inflammatory and non-inflammatory acne lesions on the face, shoulders, and upper back.
  - No nodules, cysts, or evidence of scarring.
- **Hirsutism:**
  - Mild to moderate hirsutism on the upper lip, chin, and lower abdomen (Ferriman–Gallwey score: 10).
- **Other Findings:**
  - Normal BMI: 22.5 kg/m$^2$.
  - No acanthosis nigricans, striae, or other signs of hyperandrogenism.
  - Normal thyroid gland on palpation.

## INVESTIGATIONS AND RESULTS:

1. **Hormonal Panel:**
   - **Free Testosterone:** Mildly elevated.
   - **DHEA-S:** Normal.
   - **LH/FSH Ratio:** Elevated at 3:1 (suggestive of polycystic ovary syndrome).
   - **Prolactin:** Normal.
   - **TSH:** Normal.
2. **Pelvic Ultrasound:**
   - Bilateral polycystic ovaries noted.

## WHAT IS THE DIAGNOSIS?

- **Polycystic Ovary Syndrome (PCOS)** presenting with acne and mild hirsutism.
- **Moderate Acne Vulgaris.**

PCOS is a common hormone imbalance that affects the ovaries. In the case of this patient, it is causing acne and mild hirsutism (excess hair growth on the face or body) because her body is producing slightly higher levels of male hormones (androgens) than usual. These hormones can make the skin oilier, leading to breakouts, and can also cause some extra hair growth in areas like the upper lip, chin, or lower abdomen.

PCOS can also affect the menstrual cycle, making periods irregular or delayed. It may be harder to get pregnant, but there are treatments to help if needed. Managing PCOS usually involves lifestyle changes like healthy eating and exercise, and if symptoms are bothersome, medications such as birth control pills or anti-androgen treatments can help regulate hormones, improve acne, and reduce excess hair growth.

## HOW WOULD YOU MANAGE THIS PATIENT?

1. **Lifestyle Management:**
   - Encourage a balanced diet with low-glycaemic-index foods.
   - Regular physical activity to help manage insulin resistance often associated with PCOS.
2. **Pharmacological Treatment:**
   - **First line:** Combined oral contraceptive pill (COCP) containing an anti-androgenic progestin (e.g., drospirenone) to address acne and hirsutism. Discuss safety and efficacy, particularly in relation to her upcoming marriage and potential plans for pregnancy.
   - Consider topical retinoids or benzoyl peroxide for acne management.
   - Option to add oral anti-androgens like spironolactone if COCP alone is insufficient, with contraception counselling.
3. **Cosmetic Interventions:**
   - Discuss laser hair removal or electrolysis for hirsutism.
   - Continue waxing and cosmetic measures as desired.
4. **Emotional Support:**
   - Acknowledge her concerns about appearance and upcoming wedding. Offer reassurance and timeline for expected improvement.
5. **Specialist Referral:**
   - Endocrinologist consultation if symptoms do not respond to initial management or if hormonal imbalances worsen.

### What features would suggest an underlying endocrinological issue rather than typical acne?

- Presence of **hirsutism** (upper lip, chin, lower abdomen).
- **Mildly elevated free testosterone**.
- **LH/FSH ratio 3:1** (suggestive of PCOS).
- Bilateral polycystic ovaries on ultrasound.
- Normal BMI and regular menstrual cycles – PCOS can present with mild endocrine manifestations without obvious metabolic syndrome.

### How does PCOS cause the patient's acne and hirsutism?

- Elevated androgens cause increased production of sebum, which leads to acne.
- Androgens stimulate our hair follicles, which causes hirsutism.
- Patients with this condition often have insulin resistance, which can contribute to androgen excess.

### What is the first-line pharmacological management for her PCOS-related acne and hirsutism?

- A COCP with androgenic progestin (Drospirenone). This suppresses ovarian androgen production, helping not only to regulate the menstrual cycle but also to generally improve acne and hirsutism over approximately 3–6 months.

CASE 17

# Knee Pain

## Doctor's Notes

*Patient Details:*

- **Name:** Daniel Jones
- **Age:** 28
- **Occupation:** Amateur Soccer Player
- **Presenting Complaint:** Right knee pain following a sports injury; has had an MRI scan done early last week (has not received the results yet)
- **Setting:** Family Medicine Clinic

## PATIENT'S SIMULATED SCRIPT:

### Opening Statement:

"I hurt my knee during a match last week, and it's been painful and unstable since then."

**Examiner instruction – please perform a knee examination focusing on special tests.**

## HISTORY:

- **Presenting Symptoms:**
  - Sudden onset of pain in the right knee after twisting injury during a soccer game.
  - Felt a "popping" sensation at the time of injury.
  - Knee swelling developed within hours.
  - Complains of instability and difficulty bearing weight on the affected leg.
- **Associated Symptoms:**
  - No numbness or tingling.
  - No locking but occasional catching sensation.
  - Limited range of motion due to pain.
- **Lifestyle Factors:**
  - Plays soccer regularly, involved in competitive matches.
  - No previous significant knee injuries.

## DRUG HISTORY:

- **Regular Medications:** None.
- **Allergies:** None known.
- **Recent Medications:** Took over-the-counter ibuprofen for pain relief.

## FAMILY HISTORY:

- No family history of musculoskeletal or connective tissue disorders.

## IDEAS, CONCERNS, EXPECTATIONS:

- **Ideas:** Thinks he may have damaged something in his knee due to the popping sound and ongoing instability.
- **Concerns:** Worried about long-term damage and whether he'll be able to play soccer again.
- **Expectations:** Hopes for an accurate diagnosis and treatment plan, possibly avoiding surgery.

## ON EXAMINATION:

- **General Appearance:** No signs of distress; walks with a slight limp.
- **Right Knee Examination:**
  - Swelling and mild effusion.
  - Tenderness over the lateral joint line.
  - Reduced range of motion, particularly in flexion.
  - No erythema or warmth.
  - Negative McMurray test.
- **Special Tests:**
  - **Anterior Drawer Test:** Positive; significant anterior translation of the tibia relative to the femur.
  - **Lachman Test:** Positive; increased anterior tibial movement with a soft endpoint.
  - **Pivot Shift Test:** Positive, reproducing knee instability.

## INVESTIGATIONS AND RESULTS:

1. **X-Ray of the Right Knee:** No fractures or bony abnormalities.
2. **MRI of the Right Knee:** Complete tear of the anterior cruciate ligament (ACL). No significant meniscal injury.

## WHAT IS THE DIAGNOSIS?

**Anterior Cruciate Ligament Tear.**

An ACL tear is a common knee injury that happens when the ACL, one of the key ligaments inside the knee, gets stretched or torn. The ACL helps stabilize the knee during movement, especially when stopping suddenly, changing direction, or jumping.

If one has an ACL tear, one may have felt or heard a "pop" in the knee, followed by pain, swelling, and difficulty walking or bending the knee. This type of injury is common in sports like soccer, basketball, or skiing.

Treatment depends on the severity of the tear and the patient's activity level. Mild tears may heal with physical therapy and a knee brace, but complete tears often require surgery (ACL reconstruction), especially for active individuals. After surgery, rehabilitation is needed to regain strength and movement.

## WHAT FEATURES IN THIS PATIENT'S HISTORY AND EXAMINATION SUGGEST AN ACL TEAR?

Sudden twisting injury with a popping sensation, immediate swelling, feeling of instability.

Examination findings are also supportive of an ACL tear.

### What are the indications for surgical versus nonsurgical management of an ACL tear?

- **Surgical:** Young, active/athlete wishing to return to sports involving pivoting, and those with persistent instability despite conservative therapy.
- **Non-Surgical:** Patients with sedentary lifestyle and minimal functional instability.

### What are the typical management options in a patient with this injury?

1. **Non-Surgical Management (for low-demand patients or those not playing sports):**
    - Physical therapy focusing on quadriceps and hamstring strengthening.
    - Activity modification to avoid pivoting or high-impact sports.
    - Use of a knee brace for stability during daily activities.
2. **Surgical Management (for active or high-demand patients):**
    - ACL reconstruction using autografts (hamstring or patellar tendon) or allografts.
    - Rehabilitation before surgery to strengthen surrounding muscles and optimize outcome.
3. **Post-Surgical Rehabilitation:**
    - Phase 1 (Weeks 1–4): Pain and swelling control, gentle range of motion exercises, and isometric quadriceps strengthening.
    - Phase 2 (Weeks 4–12): Progressive weight bearing, strengthening, and proprioception training.
    - Phase 3 (Months 3–6): Advanced strengthening and endurance exercises; sports-specific drills.
    - Phase 4 (6+ Months): Return to full activity and sports.

### What complications should the patient be counselled about following ACL reconstruction?

- **Early Postoperative Complications:**
    - Infection.
    - Deep vein thrombosis.
    - Persistent pain or stiffness.
- **Long-Term Complications:**
    - Graft failure or re-rupture.
    - Residual knee instability.
    - Patellar tendinitis or anterior knee pain.
    - Post-traumatic osteoarthritis.

CASE 18

# Back Pain – Ankylosing Spondylitis

## Doctor's Notes

*Patient Details:*

- **Name:** James Carter
- **Age:** 45
- **Occupation:** Construction Worker
- **Presenting Complaint:** Chronic lower back pain
- **Setting:** Family Medicine Clinic

## PATIENT'S SIMULATED SCRIPT:

### Opening Statement:

"I've had this back pain for months now, and it's just not getting any better."

## HISTORY:

- **Presenting Symptoms:**
  - Persistent lower back pain for 8 months, worse in the morning and improves with activity.
  - Stiffness in the morning lasting for over an hour.
  - Pain occasionally radiates to the buttocks bilaterally but does not go down the legs.
  - Difficulty sleeping due to pain, particularly in the second half of the night.
- **Associated Symptoms:**
  - Fatigue and weight loss (approximately 5 kg in the last 6 months).
  - Reports mild discomfort in both heels.
- **Lifestyle and Social History:**
  - Heavy smoker, smoking 20 cigarettes per day for 25 years.
  - Consumes alcohol socially, about four to five drinks per week.
  - Works long hours with frequent heavy lifting.
  - Limited exercise due to pain.

## DRUG HISTORY:

- **Regular Medications:** Occasionally takes over-the-counter ibuprofen.
- **Allergies:** None known.
- **Recent Medications:** None prescribed recently.

## FAMILY HISTORY:

- Father has hypertension, mother has rheumatoid arthritis.
- No family history of back pain.

## IDEAS, CONCERNS, EXPECTATIONS:

- **Ideas:** Thinks the pain might be due to his work or smoking affecting his back health.
- **Concerns:** Worried the pain might be permanent and impact his ability to work and provide for his family.
- **Expectations:** Hopes for pain relief and a plan to manage the condition without surgery.

## ON EXAMINATION:

- **General Appearance:** Appears fatigued and uncomfortable sitting.
- **Vitals:** BP 130/82 mmHg, HR 78 bpm, $SpO_2$ 96% on room air.
- **Back Examination:**
  - Tenderness over the sacroiliac joints bilaterally.
  - Reduced range of motion in lumbar flexion and extension.
  - Schober test: Reduced lumbar flexion with <4 cm increase in distance.
  - Normal lower limb power, sensation, and reflexes.
  - No signs of peripheral arthritis.

## INVESTIGATIONS AND RESULTS:

1. ***X-Ray of Sacroiliac Joints:*** Bilateral sacroiliitis with joint space narrowing and sclerosis.
2. ***Blood Tests:*** Elevated inflammatory markers (ESR and CRP).

## WHAT IS THE DIAGNOSIS?

**Ankylosing Spondylitis.**

Ankylosing spondylitis (AS) is a type of arthritis that mainly affects the spine, causing chronic (long-term) back pain and stiffness. It occurs because the immune system mistakenly attacks the joints in the spine, leading to inflammation and stiffness. Over time, the bones in the spine can fuse together, making movement more difficult.

Symptoms often start gradually, usually in early adulthood, with pain and stiffness in the lower back and hips, especially in the morning or after resting. Unlike regular back pain, AS improves with movement but worsens with inactivity. Some people may also have pain in the shoulders, ribs, or even eye inflammation (uveitis).

There is no cure, but treatment helps manage symptoms. This includes exercise, physical therapy, pain-relieving medications (NSAIDs), and in some cases, biologic drugs to reduce inflammation and slow disease progression. Staying active is one of the best ways to keep the spine flexible.

## OUTLINE HOW YOU WOULD MANAGE THIS PATIENT:

### Immediate Steps:

1. **Lifestyle Modifications:**
   - Strongly encourage smoking cessation, explaining its impact on systemic inflammation and disease progression.
   - Advise on maintaining a healthy weight.

2. **Medications:**
    - Start a trial of NSAIDs (e.g., naproxen) for symptom control.
    - Refer to a rheumatologist for further assessment and consideration of biologic therapy (e.g., TNF inhibitors) if symptoms persist or are severe.
3. **Physical Therapy:**
    - Refer to physiotherapy for a tailored exercise program focusing on posture correction, spinal flexibility, and core strengthening.

## Long-Term Management:

1. **Education and Support:**
    - Provide information about AS, its chronic nature, and importance of adherence to therapy.
    - Recommend joining patient support groups.
2. **Monitoring and Follow-up:**
    - Schedule regular reviews to monitor symptoms, disease progression, and medication side effects.
    - Repeat imaging and inflammatory markers as needed to assess response to treatment.

### What features would support inflammatory back pain (IBP) as opposed to mechanical back pain?

- **Type:** Inflammatory (axial) back pain.
- **Features supporting IBP:**
    - Onset <45 years (usually early adulthood).
    - Insidious onset, chronic (>3 months).
    - Morning stiffness >30 minutes.
    - Improvement with exercise/movement.
    - Worsening with rest or inactivity.
    - Night pain, especially in the second half of the night.
- **Mechanical back pain features:** Pain worsens with activity, improves with rest, usually short duration (<30 minutes morning stiffness), often age >40.
- **In this patient:** Pain is worse in the morning, improves with activity, lasts >8 months → supports IBP.

### What key clinical findings support a diagnosis of AS?

- Reduced lumbar flexion (Schober test <4 cm).
- Tenderness over sacroiliac joints.
- Morning stiffness >1 hour.
- Bilateral buttock pain.
- Heel pain (enthesitis).
- Fatigue and systemic features (weight loss).
- Positive HLA-B27.
- Elevated inflammatory markers (ESR/CRP).
- Radiographic sacroiliitis (joint space narrowing, sclerosis).

### Which investigations would you want to order to confirm the diagnosis?

- HLA-B27 testing.
- ESR and CRP (inflammatory markers).

## Imaging:

- X-ray sacroiliac joints (showing sacroiliitis).
- MRI of sacroiliac joints/spine if early disease suspected (detects inflammation before x-ray changes).

### When would we consider starting biologic therapy?

Indicated in patients with:

- Persistent active disease despite NSAIDs.
- Severe functional impairment.
- Radiographic progression.

## Options:

- TNF inhibitors (e.g., etanercept, adalimumab).
- IL-17 inhibitors (e.g., secukinumab).

# CASE 19 Psoriatic Arthritis

## Doctor's Notes

*Patient Details:*

- **Name:** Sarah Daniels
- **Age:** 35
- **Occupation:** Teacher
- **Presenting Complaint:** Right knee pain and rash
- **Setting:** Family Medicine Clinic

## PATIENT'S SIMULATED SCRIPT:

### Opening Statement:

"I've been having pain in my knee, and I also noticed this rash on my skin."

## HISTORY:

- **Presenting Symptoms:**
  - Right knee pain for the past 3 months, gradually worsening.
  - Rash on the knee and hands, noticed about 6 weeks ago. The rash is scaly and slightly itchy.
  - Swelling and stiffness in some of the fingers on both hands, particularly in the morning.
  - No history of trauma to the knee or rash.
- **Associated Symptoms:**
  - Mild fatigue.
  - Occasional low back pain.
  - No fever, chills, or recent infections.
- **Lifestyle and Social History:**
  - Non-smoker.
  - Drinks socially, two to three glasses of wine per week.
  - Engages in moderate physical activity but has reduced exercise due to knee pain.
- **Work Impact:** Difficulty standing for long periods due to knee discomfort.

## DRUG HISTORY:

- **Regular Medications:** None.
- **Allergies:** None known.
- **Recent Medications:** Over-the-counter ibuprofen for pain relief.

## FAMILY HISTORY:

- Mother diagnosed with rheumatoid arthritis in her 50s.
- No other significant family history of autoimmune conditions.

## IDEAS, CONCERNS, EXPECTATIONS:

- **Ideas:** Wonders if the rash and joint symptoms could be related.
- **Concerns:** Worries the symptoms might indicate a serious or chronic condition.
- **Expectations:** Hopes for a diagnosis and effective treatment to manage the pain and rash.

## ON EXAMINATION:

- **General Appearance:** Alert, no acute distress.
- **Vitals:** BP 118/74 mmHg, HR 78 bpm, temperature 36.8°C, $SpO_2$ 98% on room air.
- **Knee Examination:**
  - Swelling and mild warmth over the right knee.
  - Tenderness on palpation of the joint line.
  - Reduced range of motion due to pain.
  - No ligament instability.
- **Hand Examination:**
  - Swelling of the second and third digits (dactylitis) on the right hand.
  - Mild tenderness and stiffness in multiple finger joints.
- **Skin Examination:**
  - Psoriatic plaques on the right knee and extensor surfaces of both hands.
  - No nail pitting or onycholysis observed.
- **Other Findings:** Normal spine examination.

## INVESTIGATIONS AND RESULTS:

1. **Blood Tests:**
   - Elevated ESR and CRP.
   - Negative rheumatoid factor (RF) and anti-CCP antibodies.
2. **X-Ray of Right Knee:**
   - Joint space narrowing with periarticular osteopenia.
   - No fractures or dislocations.
3. **Skin Biopsy:** Consistent with psoriasis.

## WHAT IS THE MOST LIKELY DIAGNOSIS?

**Psoriatic Arthritis.**

Psoriatic arthritis (PsA) is a type of arthritis that affects some people who have psoriasis, a skin condition that causes red, scaly patches on the skin. In PsA, the immune system mistakenly attacks the joints, leading to pain, swelling, and stiffness, especially in the fingers, toes, knees, and lower back. Some people also experience fatigue and nail changes (like pitting or separation from the nail bed).

PsA can vary from mild to severe, and if left untreated, may cause permanent joint damage. Symptoms often come and go, with periods of flare-ups and remission.

## WHAT ARE THE TREATMENT OPTIONS FOR PSA?

- **NSAIDs:** Symptomatic relief of pain and inflammation.
- **DMARDs:** Methotrexate, sulfasalazine for disease-modifying therapy.
- **Biologics:** TNF inhibitors, IL-17 inhibitors for refractory disease.
- **Dermatological Care:** Topical corticosteroids, vitamin D analogs.
- **Lifestyle:** Low-impact exercise, physiotherapy, stress management.

### What non-pharmacological measures would you recommend to this patient?

- Low-impact exercise
- Weight management
- Physiotherapy for joint mobility and strength
- Stress reduction to limit psoriasis flares

### How can this condition affect long-term joint function?

- Permanent joint deformities
- Reduced range of motion
- Functional disability
- Increased risk of osteoarthritis and chronic pain

### What red flags should this patient be warned to look out for?

- Rapidly progressive joint swelling
- Severe pain unrelieved by NSAIDs
- Systemic symptoms (fever, weight loss)
- Signs of spinal involvement causing neurological deficits

CASE 20

# Heat Exhaustion

## Doctor's Notes

*Patient Details:*

- **Name:** Emily Smith
- **Age:** 32
- **Occupation:** Teacher
- **Presenting Complaint:** Sudden collapse during a hike on a hot day
- **Setting:** Family Medicine Department

## PATIENT'S SIMULATED SCRIPT:

### Opening Statement:

"I was hiking in the desert area near Sharjah when I suddenly collapsed. I felt dizzy and faint, and I couldn't continue walking. It was very hot, and I wasn't wearing a hat or sunglasses. I didn't feel any chest pain, but I was really exhausted."

## HISTORY:

The patient, a healthy 32-year-old female who reports collapsing during a hike in the summer heat. She was not wearing protective clothing such as a hat or sunglasses, and she did not carry an umbrella. The patient describes feeling dizzy, fatigued, and lightheaded, and believes she may have overexerted herself in the heat. There was no loss of consciousness, chest pain, shortness of breath, or palpitations before or after the collapse. She denies any recent illness, fever, or other significant symptoms.

## DRUG HISTORY:

- No known chronic medications.
- No recent use of over-the-counter or herbal supplements.
- Denies alcohol or substance use.

## FAMILY HISTORY:

- Non-contributory.
- No known family history of cardiovascular disease, diabetes, or metabolic disorders.

## IDEAS, CONCERNS, EXPECTATIONS:

- **Ideas:** Wonders if the collapse occurred due to not being fit enough.
- **Concerns:** She is worried about whether this collapse is a sign of a more serious condition, such as a heart issue. She is also concerned about the impact of future hikes under similar conditions.
- **Expectations:** The patient expects reassurance about her condition and clear advice on preventing a recurrence. She is hoping for some guidance on how to manage hikes safely in the future, especially in hot weather.

## ON EXAMINATION:

- **General Appearance:** Alert, oriented, and comfortable, no signs of distress at present.
- **Vital Signs:** Stable, with normal blood pressure, pulse rate, and respiratory rate.
- **Temperature:** Normal, no fever.
- **Cardiovascular:** Regular heart rate, no murmurs.
- **Respiratory:** Clear lungs on auscultation, no wheezing or crackles.
- **Neurological:** Alert and oriented, no focal neurological deficits.
- **Abdomen:** Soft, non-tender, no signs of dehydration (skin turgor normal).

## WHAT IS THE MOST LIKELY DIAGNOSIS?

**Heat Exhaustion.**

What is the differential diagnosis?

- **Heat Stroke** (needs to be ruled out due to the risk of organ damage if untreated).
- **Dehydration** causing hypotension or collapse.
- **Hypoglycaemia** from exertion without adequate food intake.
- **Electrolyte Imbalance** from excessive sweating.

**Heat stroke** is a **life-threatening condition** that happens when the body **overheats** and can no longer cool itself down. This usually occurs due to **prolonged exposure to high temperatures or intense physical activity in hot weather**. When this happens, body temperature can rise **above 104°F (40°C)**, leading to **serious damage to the brain, heart, kidneys, and muscles**.

## MANAGEMENT OPTIONS:

- **Initial Management:**
  - Move to a cool, shaded area to avoid further heat exposure.
  - Rehydrate with oral fluids (preferably electrolytes or oral rehydration solutions).
  - Apply cooling methods (cool packs, misting with water, fanning).
  - Monitor vital signs closely for the next few hours to assess stability.
- **Further Management:**
  - If symptoms persist or worsen, consider IV fluids for rehydration.
  - Monitor glucose levels to rule out hypoglycaemia.
  - Blood tests (electrolytes, kidney function) may be warranted if the patient shows signs of ongoing dehydration or electrolyte imbalances.

## FOLLOW-UP:

- **Short-term follow-up:** Ensure the patient follows up in 24–48 hours if she experiences any ongoing symptoms (e.g., weakness, dizziness).
- **Long-term follow-up:** Advise a checkup if any concerns about chronic dehydration or cardiovascular health arise.

## SAFETY NETTING:

- **Advice on future hiking:** Instruct the patient to take precautions when hiking in hot conditions (e.g., wear appropriate clothing, take frequent water breaks, avoid peak heat hours, use sunscreen).
- **Symptoms to watch for:** Return to the emergency department if any of the following symptoms occur: severe headache, confusion, chest pain, shortness of breath, or fainting.

CASE

# Skin Burn 21

## Doctor's Notes

***Patient Details:***

- **Name:** Sally Roberts
- **Age:** 35
- **Occupation:** Chef
- **Presenting Complaint:** Burn to the right hand
- **Setting:** Primary Care Clinic

## PATIENT'S SIMULATED SCRIPT:

### Opening Statement:

"I burned my right hand while cooking. It's very painful, and I noticed some blisters."

## HISTORY:

The patient reports that the burn occurred earlier today while handling a hot pan. The affected area is the palm and fingers of the right hand. Pain was severe initially but has lessened slightly. The patient immediately ran the hand under cold water for 15 minutes but did not apply any creams. There are visible blisters, and some areas feel raw. There is no numbness or loss of movement in the fingers. No other injuries were sustained.

## DRUG HISTORY:

- **Regular Medications:** None.
- **Allergies:** Penicillin.

## FAMILY HISTORY:

- Non-contributory.

## IDEAS, CONCERNS, EXPECTATIONS:

- **Ideas:** The patient thinks the burn is moderate and may require medical care to heal properly.
- **Concerns:** The patient is worried about infection, pain management, and whether the burn will lead to long-term scarring or impaired hand function.
- **Expectations:** The patient expects wound care, pain relief, and advice on ensuring proper healing and preventing complications.

## WHAT WOULD YOUR EXAMINATION COMPRISE FOR THIS TYPE OF PATIENT?

### General Assessment:

- **General appearance:** Assess the patient's overall condition and level of distress.
- **Vitals:** Check for signs of systemic involvement (e.g., tachycardia, hypotension, fever) that might suggest a severe burn or infection.

### Inspection of the Burn Area:

- **Location:** Identify the specific areas affected (e.g., palm, dorsum, fingers).
- **Extent:** Estimate the total body surface area (TBSA) affected using tools like the **Rule of Nines** (for larger burns) or the patient's palm (approximately 1% TBSA).
- **Depth:** Assess burn depth based on appearance:
  - **Superficial (1st degree):** Red, dry, painful.
  - **Partial thickness (2nd degree):** Red or pink, blisters, moist, painful.
  - **Full thickness (3rd degree):** White, leathery, or charred; no pain in the burned area (due to nerve damage).
- **Blisters:** Note the presence, size, and condition of blisters (intact or ruptured).
- **Edges:** Look for signs of spreading erythema or discoloration, which may indicate infection or a secondary process.
- **Signs of Infection:** Assess for pus, foul odour, increased redness, or swelling beyond the burn edges.

### Functional Assessment:

- **Range of Motion (ROM):** Evaluate active and passive movement of all joints in the hand (fingers, thumb, wrist) to identify stiffness or pain.
- **Grip Strength:** Assess for functional deficits in the grip and pinch.

### Sensory Examination:

- Test for sensation in the affected and surrounding areas to assess nerve involvement:
  - **Light touch:** Use a cotton swab or light stroke.
  - **Pinprick:** Check for pain response.
  - **Temperature:** Evaluate the ability to sense hot and cold.
  - **Two-point discrimination:** Check fine sensory function if deeper injuries are suspected.

### Circulation Assessment:

- **Capillary Refill:** Press on the nail bed or a fingertip and observe capillary refill time (<2 seconds is normal).
- **Peripheral Pulses:** Palpate radial and ulnar pulses to assess arterial circulation.
- **Colour and Temperature:** Note skin temperature and colour in and around the burn area to rule out ischaemia.
- **Swelling/Compartment Syndrome:** Check for tightness or increased pressure in the hand or digits, which can compromise circulation.

### Assessment of Surrounding Areas:

- Examine adjacent skin and structures for any secondary injuries or burns.
- Look for associated injuries (e.g., cuts, abrasions) that may have occurred during the incident.

### Systemic Examination:

- For severe burns or concerns of inhalation injury, expand the examination to assess for systemic complications:
  - **Respiratory:** Check for airway involvement if there is a history of exposure to flame or smoke.
  - **Hydration:** Look for signs of dehydration if the burn is extensive.

## ON EXAMINATION:

- **General Appearance:** Alert, no signs of distress.
- **Right Hand:**
  - Redness, swelling, and tenderness over the palm and fingers.
  - Multiple large blisters, some intact, others ruptured, with exposed dermis visible.
  - The skin around the blisters is erythematous but not extending significantly beyond the burn area.
  - No signs of infection (no pus, fever, or streaking).
  - Sensation is intact, and motor function is normal.
  - Capillary refill is normal, indicating good peripheral circulation.

## WHAT IS THE MOST LIKELY DIAGNOSIS?

**Second-Degree Burn (Partial-Thickness Burn).**

A partial thickness burn is a type of burn injury that affects both the outer layer of the skin (epidermis) and part of the deeper layer (dermis). It is more serious than a superficial burn (like a mild sunburn) but not as severe as a full-thickness burn, which destroys all skin layers.

There are two types of partial-thickness burns:

1. Superficial partial thickness burns – Affect the top part of the dermis. The skin looks red, blistered, moist, and very painful. Healing usually takes 1–2 weeks with minimal scarring.
2. Deep partial thickness burns – Affect the deeper part of the dermis. The skin may look white, blotchy, or have less sensation because of nerve damage. Healing takes more than 2 weeks and may leave scars or require treatment like skin grafting.

Treatment includes cleaning the wound, applying dressings, pain management, and keeping the skin moisturized. Severe burns may need specialist care to prevent infection and improve healing.

## HOW WOULD YOU MANAGE THIS PATIENT?

1. **Immediate Management:**
   - **Wound Care:**
     - Clean the affected area with cool saline or clean water to remove debris.
     - Leave intact blisters undisturbed. For ruptured blisters, debride dead tissue if necessary under sterile conditions.
   - **Topical Treatment:**
     - Apply silver sulfadiazine cream (if not contraindicated) to the affected area. Alternatively, use a non-stick dressing with a petroleum-based ointment to keep the wound moist.
   - **Pain Management:**
     - Prescribe paracetamol or ibuprofen for pain relief. If the pain is severe, consider short-term prescription analgesics.
   - **Dressings:**
     - Cover the burn with a sterile, non-adherent dressing. Change dressings daily or as needed, ensuring a clean, moist healing environment.
2. **Further Management:**
   - Administer a **tetanus booster** if the patient's vaccination status is unclear or not up to date.
   - If the burn covers a significant portion of the hand or shows signs of potential infection, refer the patient to a burn specialist.

3. **Patient Education:**
   - Avoid popping intact blisters, as they act as a natural barrier against infection.
   - Elevate the hand to reduce swelling.
   - Avoid using home remedies or unverified treatments (e.g., butter, toothpaste).

# CASE 22 Hypertension (Non-Compliant)

## Doctor's Notes

*Patient Details:*

- **Name:** Huvad Varik
- **Age:** 52
- **Occupation:** Accountant
- **Presenting Complaint:** Uncontrolled high blood pressure
- **Setting:** Primary Care Clinic

## PATIENT'S SIMULATED SCRIPT:

### Opening Statement:

"My blood pressure has been very high even though I'm taking all my medications regularly. I'm feeling lightheaded and tired, and I'm worried something serious might happen."

## HISTORY:

The patient is a 52-year-old male with a 10-year history of hypertension. He has been prescribed three medications: lisinopril 20 mg, amlodipine 10 mg, and hydrochlorothiazide 25 mg daily. Despite adherence to his treatment regimen, his blood pressure remains uncontrolled. He reports occasional headaches, dizziness, and mild fatigue. There is no chest pain, palpitations, or shortness of breath. Lifestyle factors include a sedentary job, minimal exercise, and a diet high in salt and processed foods. He denies alcohol or tobacco use.

## DRUG HISTORY:

- **Regular Medications:** Lisinopril 20 mg daily, amlodipine 10 mg daily, hydrochlorothiazide 25 mg daily.
- **Allergies:** None known.

## FAMILY HISTORY:

- Father had hypertension and died of a stroke at 60.
- Mother has diabetes and hypertension.

## IDEAS, CONCERNS, EXPECTATIONS:

- **Ideas:** The patient thinks his medications have stopped working for him and he might need different ones.
- **Concerns:** He is worried about the risk of stroke or heart attack due to persistently high blood pressure.
- **Expectations:** The patient expects a solution to lower his blood pressure and advice on preventing long-term complications.

## ON EXAMINATION:

- **General Appearance:** Alert, overweight, no signs of acute distress.
- **Vitals:** BP 180/110 mmHg (measured in both arms), HR 82 bpm, regular, respiratory rate 16 bpm, temperature 36.9°C.
- **Cardiovascular Examination:**
  - Normal heart sounds, no murmurs or gallops.
  - No peripheral oedema.
- **Respiratory Examination:**
  - Clear lungs, no wheezing or crackles.
- **Neurological Examination:**
  - No focal deficits, no signs of acute stroke.

## WHAT IS THE MOST LIKELY DIAGNOSIS?

**Resistant Hypertension** – Blood pressure remains uncontrolled despite adherence to three antihypertensive medications, including a diuretic.

Resistant hypertension is high blood pressure that remains uncontrolled despite taking at least three different blood pressure medications, including a diuretic (water pill), at the correct doses. In some cases, a fourth medication may be needed to bring blood pressure under control.

This condition can occur due to several reasons, including:

- **Lifestyle factors** (such as high salt intake, obesity, or lack of exercise)
- **Other medical conditions** (such as kidney disease, sleep apnoea, or hormonal imbalances)
- **Medication issues** (not taking medications correctly or drug interactions)

Since resistant hypertension increases the risk of heart disease, stroke, and kidney problems, it is important to find and treat the underlying cause. Doctors usually recommend a combination of lifestyle changes, adjusting medications, and checking for secondary causes of high blood pressure.

## HOW WOULD YOU MANAGE THIS PATIENT?

1. **Immediate Management:**
   - **Add a fourth medication:** Spironolactone 25 mg daily is recommended for resistant hypertension unless contraindicated. Monitor potassium levels and renal function closely.
   - Consider beta-blockers (e.g., bisoprolol) or alpha-blockers (e.g., doxazosin) if spironolactone is unsuitable.
2. **Further Evaluation:**
   - Investigate secondary causes of hypertension:
     - **Renal artery stenosis:** Perform a renal ultrasound or Doppler.

- **Primary hyperaldosteronism**: Check plasma aldosterone and renin levels.
- **Obstructive sleep apnoea**: Assess sleep patterns and consider a sleep study.
- **Thyroid dysfunction**: Check thyroid function tests.

- Perform a 24-hour ambulatory blood pressure monitoring to rule out white-coat hypertension.

3. **Lifestyle Modifications:**
   - **Diet:** Implement the DASH diet (explained below).
   - **Physical Activity:** Encourage at least 150 minutes of moderate-intensity exercise per week.
   - **Salt Restriction:** Limit sodium intake to less than 2300 mg per day, ideally aiming for 100 mg per day.
   - **Weight Loss:** Set realistic goals for gradual weight loss if the patient is overweight.
4. **Patient Education:**
   - Emphasize the importance of lifestyle changes as a cornerstone of blood pressure management.
   - Discuss the chronic nature of hypertension and the need for regular follow-up and medication adjustments.

## FOLLOW-UP:

- Review in 2 weeks to assess response to the medication adjustment.
- Monitor blood pressure, renal function, and potassium levels.

## HOW TO TREAT HYPERTENSIVE URGENCY

- **Definition:** Hypertensive urgency is defined as a systolic BP ≥180 mmHg or diastolic BP ≥110 mmHg without evidence of acute end-organ damage.
- **Treatment Goals:** Gradual reduction in blood pressure over 24–48 hours to avoid hypotension and associated complications.
- **Medications**:
  - **Oral agents** are typically sufficient:
    - **Captopril** (25 mg): Reduces BP within 15–30 minutes.
    - **Clonidine** (0.1–0.2 mg): Effective within 30 minutes to 2 hours.
    - **Amlodipine** (5–10 mg): Offers steady BP reduction.
  - Avoid excessive lowering of BP (no more than 25% within the first 24 hours).

## WHAT IS THE DASH DIET?

The **Dietary Approaches to Stop Hypertension (DASH)** diet is a nutritional plan designed to lower blood pressure by emphasizing heart-healthy foods and limiting sodium intake.

### Key Components:

1. **Fruits and Vegetables**
   - Aim for four to five servings of each per day.
   - Examples: Bananas, oranges, spinach, broccoli.
2. **Whole Grains**
   - Consume six to eight servings per day.
   - Examples: Brown rice, whole wheat bread, oatmeal.
3. **Low-Fat Dairy**
   - Include two to three servings per day.
   - Examples: Skim milk, low-fat yogurt, cheese.
4. **Lean Protein**
   - Limit to two or fewer servings per day.
   - Examples: Chicken, fish, tofu.

5. **Nuts, Seeds, and Legumes**
   - Include four to five servings per week.
   - Examples: Almonds, beans, lentils.
6. **Fats and Oils**
   - Limit total fat intake and focus on healthy fats like olive oil.
7. **Sweets and Added Sugars**
   - Allow no more than five servings per week.

## Sodium Restriction:

- Target less than 2300 mg of sodium daily (ideally 1500 mg).
- Avoid processed foods, canned soups, and salty snacks.

## Benefits:

- The DASH diet can lower systolic blood pressure by 8–14 mmHg and improve cardiovascular health when combined with physical activity.

**What advice would you give regarding complications and prognosis?**

Poorly controlled hypertension increases risk of:

- Stroke (especially haemorrhagic)
- Ischaemic heart disease and heart failure
- Chronic kidney disease
- Retinopathy

With good control, risk reduction is substantial (e.g., lowering SBP by 10 mmHg reduces stroke risk by ~40%).

# CASE 23 Botulinum Toxicity

## Doctor's Notes

*Patient Details:*

- **Name:** Venu Muus
- **Age:** 35
- **Occupation:** Chef
- **Presenting Complaint:** Difficulty swallowing, double vision, and generalized weakness
- **Setting:** Emergency Department

## PATIENT'S SIMULATED SCRIPT:

### Opening Statement:

"I've been feeling weak all over, and now I'm having trouble swallowing. My vision is blurry, and I see double sometimes."

## HISTORY:

The patient is a 35-year-old male who developed symptoms 24 hours after attending a private dinner party where homemade canned foods (vegetables and fish) were served. He reports experiencing nausea and dry mouth initially, which progressed to difficulty swallowing, slurred speech, and double vision. He also describes generalized weakness that worsened over time, making it difficult to walk. No fever, chest pain, or shortness of breath was reported.

## DRUG HISTORY:

- **Regular Medications:** None.
- **Allergies:** None known.

## FAMILY HISTORY:

- Non-contributory.

## IDEAS, CONCERNS, EXPECTATIONS:

- **Ideas:** The patient believes the symptoms might be related to the food consumed at the dinner party.
- **Concerns:** He is worried about the possibility of a severe or irreversible condition affecting his nervous system.
- **Expectations:** The patient expects a diagnosis and urgent treatment to address his worsening symptoms.

## ON EXAMINATION:

- **General Appearance:** Alert but visibly fatigued and weak.
- **Vitals:** BP 110/70 mmHg, HR 80 bpm, regular, RR 18 bpm, temperature 36.7°C, oxygen saturation 97% on room air.
- **Neurological Examination:**
  - **Cranial Nerves:**
    - Ptosis bilaterally, diminished pupillary response to light, diplopia.
    - Dysarthria and dysphagia.
  - **Motor Function:**
    - Generalized muscle weakness, more pronounced in proximal muscles.
    - No sensory deficits.
  - **Reflexes:**
    - Diminished deep tendon reflexes.
- **Respiratory System:**
- Normal breath sounds, no evidence of respiratory distress; however, observe closely for potential respiratory muscle involvement.

## WHAT IS THE MOST LIKELY DIAGNOSIS?

**Botulinum Toxicity** – suspected due to the history of consuming potentially contaminated canned food and the clinical presentation of descending paralysis, cranial nerve involvement, and autonomic dysfunction.

Botulinum toxicity, also known as botulism, is a rare but serious condition caused by a toxin produced by the bacteria *Clostridium botulinum*. This toxin affects the nerves and leads to muscle paralysis, which can become life-threatening if it spreads to the muscles that control breathing.

## MANAGEMENT OPTIONS:

1. **Immediate Management:**
   - **Hospital Admission:** Transfer to an intensive care unit (ICU) for close monitoring of respiratory function.
   - **Antitoxin Administration:** Administer botulinum antitoxin as soon as possible to halt further progression of symptoms. The antitoxin does not reverse existing paralysis but prevents worsening.
     - Obtain the antitoxin from authorized sources (local health department or poison control centre).
2. **Respiratory Support:**
   - Monitor oxygen saturation and respiratory rate closely.
   - Be prepared for mechanical ventilation if respiratory failure occurs due to diaphragmatic paralysis.
3. **Gastrointestinal Decontamination:**
   - If within hours of ingestion, consider gastric lavage or activated charcoal (rarely indicated given the delayed onset of symptoms).
4. **Supportive Care:**
   - Intravenous fluids to maintain hydration.
   - Nutritional support, including nasogastric feeding if swallowing difficulty persists.
5. **Diagnostic Tests:**
   - **Serum Testing:** Confirm botulinum toxin by testing the patient's serum, stool, or suspected food samples.
   - **Electromyography (EMG):** May show characteristic findings of botulinum toxicity.

6. **Patient Education and Counselling:**
   - Explain the seriousness of the condition and the importance of early treatment.
   - Discuss the need for prolonged recovery and possible physical therapy to regain muscle strength.

**What is the role of botulinum antitoxin in treatment, and what are the key considerations before administration?**

- **Role:** Neutralise circulating toxin preventing neuromuscular blockade. Preexisting paralysis is not reversed; however, antitoxin should be given as soon as possible.
- **Key Considerations:**
  - Monitor for anaphylaxis during the infusion.
  - Antitoxin must be sourced from government hospitals/signpost patients to government hospitals (not usually available in private hospitals in the UAE)
  - History of horse protein hypersensitivity = likely contraindication to antitoxin.

**What advice would you give family members/partners about the patient?**

- **Signs to watch for:** Educate family members on signs of respiratory distress, such as shortness of breath or worsening weakness, requiring immediate attention.
- Advise close contacts to seek medical evaluation if they consumed the same food and show any symptoms of botulism.

**Who should you notify?**

- **Poison Control Centre:** Promptly inform the poison control centre to report the suspected case, and request guidance on obtaining the antitoxin.
- **Local Health Authorities:** Botulism is a notifiable disease due to its public health implications. Inform the relevant health department to initiate an investigation of the food source, prevent further cases, and address any public health risks.

# CASE 24 Stroke

## Doctor's Notes

*Patient Details:*

- **Name:** Ahmed Al-Bakri
- **Age:** 72
- **Occupation:** Retired teacher
- **Presenting Complaint:** Sudden onset of facial drooping and weakness
- **Setting:** Emergency Room

## PATIENT'S SIMULATED SCRIPT:

### Opening Statement:

"My face feels numb, and I can't move it properly."

## HISTORY:

- **Presenting Symptoms:**
  - Sudden onset of right-sided facial drooping that began 2 hours ago.
  - Weakness in the right arm and difficulty gripping objects.
  - Slurred speech and difficulty pronouncing words clearly.
  - No loss of consciousness or confusion.
- **Associated Symptoms:**
  - Mild headache, non-throbbing, located on the left side.
  - No nausea, vomiting, or vision changes.
  - No seizures or episodes of fainting.

## PAST MEDICAL HISTORY:

- Hypertension for 15 years.
- Type 2 diabetes mellitus for 10 years.

- Hyperlipidaemia for 8 years.
- No prior history of stroke or transient ischaemic attacks (TIAs).

## DRUG HISTORY:

- **Regular Medications:** Amlodipine 10 mg once daily, metformin 500 mg twice daily, atorvastatin 20 mg once daily.
- **Allergies:** None known.

## FAMILY HISTORY:

- Father had a stroke at the age of 70.
- Mother had hypertension.

## LIFESTYLE AND SOCIAL HISTORY:

- Non-smoker.
- Rarely consumes alcohol.
- Sedentary lifestyle with limited physical activity.
- Diet includes high carbohydrate intake and low fruit and vegetable consumption.

## IDEAS, CONCERNS, EXPECTATIONS:

- **Ideas:** Thinks he's having a bad migraine, because he feels terrible.
- **Concerns:** Worries it might be something more serious like a brain tumour.
- **Expectations:** Hopes for immediate treatment to restore normal function and prevent worsening.

## ON EXAMINATION:

- **General Appearance:** Alert but visibly distressed.
- **Vitals:** BP: 165/98 mmHg, HR: 88 bpm, regular, temperature 36.8°C, $SpO_2$: 97% on room air.
- **Neurological Examination:**
  - **Cranial Nerves:**
    - Right-sided facial drooping (lower motor neuron type).
    - Slurred speech but intact comprehension.
  - **Motor System:**
    - Right upper and lower limb weakness (Grade 3/5).
    - Left side strength normal (Grade 5/5).
  - **Reflexes:**
    - Hyperreflexia on the right side.
    - Babinski sign positive on the right.
  - **Sensation:** Reduced on the right side of the body.
  - **Coordination:** Difficulty performing finger-to-nose test with the right hand.
- **Cardiovascular Examination:** No murmurs or arrhythmias.

## INVESTIGATIONS AND RESULTS:

1. **Immediate CT Brain:** Hypodense area in the left middle cerebral artery (MCA) territory consistent with an ischaemic stroke.
2. **Blood Tests:**
   - **Random Blood Glucose:** 8.2 mmol/L
   - **HbA1c:** 7.8%

   - **Lipid Profile:** Elevated LDL (3.6 mmol/L), total cholesterol 6.2 mmol/L.
   - **INR:** 1.0
3. **ECG:** Normal sinus rhythm with no evidence of atrial fibrillation.
4. **Carotid Doppler (pending):** Ordered to assess for carotid stenosis.

## WHAT IS THE DIAGNOSIS?

**Ischaemic Stroke** affecting the left MCA territory.

An ischaemic stroke occurs when a blood clot or blockage stops blood flow to a part of the brain. This prevents oxygen from reaching brain cells, causing them to start dying within minutes. It is the most common type of stroke, making up about 85% of all strokes.

## ASIDE FROM A CT BRAIN, WHAT OTHER IMMEDIATE INVESTIGATIONS IN A SUSPECTED STROKE SHOULD BE ORDERED PRIOR TO STARTING TREATMENT?

- **Blood glucose:** hypoglycaemia may mimic stroke.
- **Full blood count, renal function, coagulation profile (INR, PT, aPTT, platelets):** essential before thrombolysis.
- **ECG:** detect atrial fibrillation or arrhythmia.
- **Cardiac enzymes:** if MI suspected.
- **Oxygen saturation, vitals:** to assess stability.
- **Further (not immediate): carotid Doppler, echocardiography, lipid profile, HbA1c** for secondary prevention.

## WHAT COMPLICATIONS OR RED FLAGS SHOULD BE CONSIDERED IN AN ACUTE STROKE PATIENT?

- **Neurological deterioration:** haemorrhagic transformation, cerebral oedema, raised ICP.
- **Respiratory compromise:** aspiration pneumonia (due to dysphagia), hypoventilation.
- **Cardiac complications:** arrhythmias, MI.
- **Venous thromboembolism:** due to immobility.
- **Pressure sores, urinary tract infections:** from bed rest.
- **Seizures:** post-stroke epilepsy.

## WHAT ARE THE GENERAL MANAGEMENT STEPS FOR A PATIENT LIKE THIS?

*Immediate Steps:*

1. **Acute Stroke Management:**
   - Administer thrombolysis with tissue plasminogen activator (tPA) if within the 4.5-hour window and no contraindications.
   - If thrombolysis is not indicated, provide antiplatelet therapy (e.g., aspirin 300 mg).
2. **Supportive Care:**
   - Monitor in a high-dependency or stroke unit for the first 24–48 hours.
   - Ensure adequate hydration and nutrition.

*Discuss the long-term secondary prevention strategies for this patient once stable:*

1. **Antiplatelet Therapy:** Aspirin 75–100 mg daily or clopidogrel if aspirin-intolerant. Dual antiplatelet for 3 weeks if minor stroke/TIA, then single.
2. **Statin Therapy:** High-intensity atorvastatin 80 mg daily (LDL target <1.8 mmol/L).
3. **Blood Pressure Control:** Optimise antihypertensives, target <140/90 mmHg (ACE inhibitors, diuretics).
4. **Diabetes Management:** Tight glycaemic control (HbA1c <7%).

5. **Lifestyle Modification:** Mediterranean diet, salt restriction, regular exercise, weight management, alcohol limitation.
6. **Screening and Treating Atrial Fibrillation:** Anticoagulation if AF detected.
7. **Carotid Intervention:** Consider endarterectomy/stenting if ≥70% stenosis in symptomatic carotid artery.

## FOLLOW-UP:

- **Neurology Referral:** For long-term management and monitoring.
- **Physical and Speech Therapy:** For rehabilitation of motor and speech functions.
- **Diabetes Management:** Adjust treatment to improve glycaemic control.

CASE 25

# Nosebleed

## Doctor's Notes

*Patient Details:*

- **Name:** Ahmed Hassan
- **Age:** 55
- **Occupation:** Accountant
- **Presenting Complaint:** Nosebleed (epistaxis)
- **Setting:** Family Medicine Clinic

## PATIENT'S SIMULATED SCRIPT:

### Opening Statement:

"My nose has been bleeding on and off for the past 2 days."

## HISTORY:

- **Presenting Symptoms:**
  - Spontaneous nosebleeds, mainly from the left nostril, lasting 5–10 minutes before stopping on their own.
  - Blood is bright red and flows easily.
  - No trauma or nasal picking reported.
  - Mild nasal dryness noticed recently.
- **Associated Symptoms:**
  - Occasional mild headache.
  - No fever, bruising, gum bleeding, or haematuria.

## PAST MEDICAL HISTORY:

- History of deep vein thrombosis (DVT) 8 months ago, on long-term anticoagulation therapy.
- Controlled hypertension diagnosed 5 years ago.

## DRUG HISTORY:

- **Regular Medications:** Warfarin 5 mg daily (INR checked regularly), amlodipine 10 mg daily for hypertension.
- **Occasional:** Paracetamol occasionally for headaches.
- **Allergies:** None known.

## FAMILY HISTORY:

- Father had a stroke at 65 years old.
- No family history of bleeding disorders.

## LIFESTYLE AND SOCIAL HISTORY:

- Smokes five to six cigarettes daily for 20 years.
- Drinks one to two cups of coffee per day, no alcohol use.
- Sedentary lifestyle with limited physical activity.

## IDEAS, CONCERNS, EXPECTATIONS:

- **Ideas:** Thinks the nosebleed might be due to dry weather or medication side effects.
- **Concerns:** Worried the nosebleed might indicate a serious issue like a blood clotting problem or a stroke risk.
- **Expectations:** Hopes to control the bleeding and ensure it's not a sign of a dangerous condition.

## ON EXAMINATION:

- **General Appearance:** Stable, not in acute distress.
- **Vitals:** BP 132/78 mmHg, HR 82 bpm, regular, temperature 36.8°C, $SpO_2$: 97% on room air.
- **ENT Examination:**
  - Active bleeding seen from the left anterior nasal septum (Kiesselbach plexus).
  - No septal perforation or significant crusting.
  - No nasal polyps or masses.
  - Oral mucosa and oropharynx unremarkable.
- **Other Systemic Examination:**
  - No petechiae, ecchymoses, or signs of systemic bleeding.
  - Chest and abdominal exams are normal.

## INVESTIGATIONS AND RESULTS:

1. **Blood Tests:**
   - **INR:** 4.2 (elevated, therapeutic range for DVT: 2–3).
   - **Hb:** 13.8 g/dL (normal).
   - **Platelet count:** 210,000/$mm^3$ (normal).
   - **Renal:** Normal renal and liver function tests.
2. **Nasal Endoscopy (if available):**
   - Bleeding localized to the anterior nasal septum without underlying masses or lesions.

## WHAT IS THE CAUSE OF THE NOSEBLEEDS?

Epistaxis secondary to over-anticoagulation from warfarin.

## HOW WOULD YOU MANAGE THIS PATIENT INITIALLY?

### Immediate Management:

1. **Stop Active Bleeding:**
   - Apply direct pressure to the nostrils by pinching them together for 10–15 minutes.
   - Administer topical vasoconstrictor (e.g., oxymetazoline spray) to reduce bleeding.
   - Cauterize the bleeding site with silver nitrate if bleeding persists after conservative measures.
2. **Anticoagulation Reversal:**
   - Administer vitamin K (1–5 mg orally or intravenously, depending on severity) to reverse the effect of warfarin.
   - Consider prothrombin complex concentrate (PCC) or fresh frozen plasma (FFP) in severe or life-threatening bleeding.
3. **Review Medications:**
   - Withhold warfarin temporarily and monitor INR closely.

**What parts of the history would you aim to explore to identify and understand the cause of the recurrent nosebleeds?**

- Local trauma (nose picking, forceful sneezing, recent nasal instrumentation).
- Nasal dryness or environmental factors.
- Use of anticoagulants (warfarin, DOACs), antiplatelets, or NSAIDs.
- History of systemic bleeding disorders (haemophilia, von Willebrand disease).
- Hypertension, liver disease, renal disease.
- Family history of bleeding or clotting disorders.
- Symptoms suggesting tumours or vascular malformations (persistent unilateral bleeding, obstruction).

**Which red flags in the history would suggest are more significant or serious cause for the nosebleeds?**

- Recurrent unilateral bleeding not related to trauma or dryness.
- Persistent bleeding despite first aid measures.
- Associated systemic symptoms (easy bruising, haematuria, gum bleeding).
- Weight loss, nasal obstruction, facial pain, or anosmia (could suggest malignancy).

**How would you manage anticoagulation in such a patient post bleed?**

- Temporarily withhold warfarin until INR returns to therapeutic range.
- Administer vitamin K if bleeding is significant.
- Reassess the target INR and adjust warfarin dosing.
- Consider alternative anticoagulants only after consulting haematology if recurrent supratherapeutic INR occurs.
- Reinforce adherence and consistency with diet and drug interactions.

**What lifestyle advice would be beneficial in reducing future nosebleeds?**

- Humidify indoor environment to prevent nasal dryness.
- Avoid nasal trauma (nose picking, aggressive blowing).
- Smoking cessation.
- Maintain consistent dietary vitamin K intake.
- Regular INR monitoring and adherence to warfarin

**What is the antidote for warfarin?**

- Vitamin K is the antidote, administered orally or intravenously based on severity.
- Prothrombin complex concentrate (PCC) or fresh frozen plasma (FFP) is used in severe or life-threatening bleeding.

# CASE 26
# Fibroids

## Doctor's Notes

*Patient Details:*

- **Name:** Amina Khalid
- **Age:** 42
- **Occupation:** School teacher
- **Presenting Complaint:** Follow-up for ultrasound and blood test results
- **Setting:** Family Medicine Clinic

## PATIENT'S SIMULATED SCRIPT:

### Opening Statement:

"I'm here to discuss the results of my tests."

## HISTORY:

- **Reason for Tests (if asked):**
  - Menorrhagia for the past 12 months, with heavy periods lasting 7–10 days, requiring frequent pad changes.
  - No post-menopausal bleeding.
- **Associated Symptoms:**
  - Fatigue and occasional light-headedness.
  - No weight loss or abdominal pain.

## PAST MEDICAL HISTORY:

- Menorrhagia, no known underlying condition identified so far.
- No history of clotting disorders or previous surgeries.

## DRUG HISTORY:

- **Medications:** Multivitamins occasionally.
- **Regular Medications:** No prescribed medications.
- **Allergies:** No known drug allergies.

## FAMILY HISTORY:

- Mother had a hysterectomy at 50 for uterine fibroids.
- Father has type 2 diabetes.

## LIFESTYLE AND SOCIAL HISTORY:

- Non-smoker, occasional tea drinker.
- Regular exercise: brisk walking three to four times a week.
- Balanced diet but admits to craving sweets recently.

## IDEAS, CONCERNS, EXPECTATIONS:

- **Ideas:** Suspects the heavy periods may be genetic.
- **Concerns:** Worries the ultrasound may have revealed something serious like cancer.
- **Expectations:** Hopes for a clear diagnosis and a treatment plan to stop the heavy bleeding.

## ON EXAMINATION:

- **General Appearance:** Alert but appears fatigued.
- **Vitals:** BP 128/78 mmHg, HR 88 bpm, regular, temperature 36.7°C, $SpO_2$ 98% on room air.
- **Abdominal Examination:**
    - Soft, non-tender.
    - No palpable masses.
    - No hepatosplenomegaly.
- **Pelvic Examination (if done or mentioned):**
    - Deferred or unremarkable if done earlier.

## INVESTIGATIONS AND RESULTS:

1. **Pelvic Ultrasound Scan:**
    - Uterus enlarged with multiple uterine fibroids. Largest fibroid is 5 cm, submucosal.
    - Endometrial thickness: 12 mm.
    - No adnexal masses or free fluid in the pelvis.
2. **Blood Tests:**
    - **Hb:** 10.2 g/dL (low, suggestive of iron deficiency anaemia).
    - **MCV:** 72 fL (low, microcytic anaemia).
    - **Serum Ferritin:** 8 ng/mL (low).
    - **Fasting Glucose:** 6.3 mmol/L (pre-diabetic range).
    - **Renal:** Normal renal and liver function tests.

## WHAT IS THE DIAGNOSIS?

1. **Uterine Fibroids** (likely causing menorrhagia).
2. **Iron Deficiency Anaemia** secondary to menorrhagia.
3. **Pre-Diabetes.**

Fibroids are noncancerous growths that develop in or around the uterus (womb). They are made of muscle and fibrous tissue and can vary in size, from as small as a seed to as large as a melon. Many women have fibroids without symptoms, but some may experience issues.

## OUTLINE HOW YOU WOULD MANAGE THIS PATIENT:

*Immediate Steps:*

1. **Address Menorrhagia and Fibroids:**
    - Refer to gynaecology for further assessment and management options such as:
        - Hormonal therapy (e.g., oral contraceptive pills, progestin IUD).
        - Biopsy, as endometrial thickness is a concern.
        - Non-hormonal options like tranexamic acid or NSAIDs for heavy bleeding.
        - Surgical options, if indicated, such as myomectomy or uterine artery embolization.
2. **Treat Iron Deficiency Anaemia:**
    - Start oral iron supplements (e.g., ferrous sulphate 325 mg once daily).
    - Encourage a diet rich in iron (e.g., red meat, green leafy vegetables, beans) and vitamin C to enhance absorption.
3. **Address Pre-Diabetes:**
    - Counsel on lifestyle modifications, including dietary adjustments to reduce sugar and refined carbohydrates.
    - Encourage regular exercise to improve glycaemic control (e.g., brisk walking 30 minutes daily).
    - Schedule a follow-up for HbA1c and glucose monitoring in 3 months.

*Long-Term Management:*

- Monitor haemoglobin levels to assess improvement.
- Regular gynaecological follow-up to manage fibroids and prevent complications.
- Annual diabetes screening and ongoing dietary counselling.

## QUESTIONS:

1. **What are the common symptoms of uterine fibroids?**
    - Heavy menstrual bleeding (menorrhagia), pelvic pressure, or pain.
    - Frequent urination or constipation if fibroids press on adjacent organs.
2. **What dietary advice can help with pre-diabetes?**
    - Reduce intake of sugary foods and beverages.
    - Focus on whole grains, lean proteins, and vegetables.
    - Regularly spaced meals to maintain blood sugar levels.
3. **When should we be concerned about endometrial thickness?**
    - If associated with abnormal uterine bleeding, such as menorrhagia in this case. Thickness up to 14 mm can be normal in a premenopausal woman if not combined with abnormal bleeding.
4. **What are the first-line medical management options for menorrhagia caused by fibroids?**
    - **Hormonal therapy:**
        - Combined oral contraceptives to regulate and reduce bleeding.
        - Levonorgestrel-releasing intrauterine device (IUD) to reduce menstrual blood loss.
    - **Non-hormonal therapy:**
        - Tranexamic acid during menses.
        - NSAIDs to reduce blood loss and relieve dysmenorrhea.
5. **What surgical options are available for uterine fibroids, and what factors influence the choice?**
    - **Myomectomy:** Preferred if fertility preservation desired.
    - **Hysterectomy:** Definitive treatment in women who have completed childbearing.
    - **Uterine Artery Embolization:** Minimally invasive, preserves the uterus but may affect fertility.
    - **Endometrial Ablation:** For small, submucosal fibroids and not desiring fertility.

# CASE 27

# UTI in Pregnancy

## Doctor's Notes

*Patient Details:*

- **Name:** Huda Saleh
- **Age:** 28
- **Occupation:** Office worker
- **Presenting Complaint:** Follow-up for antenatal care, complaints of dysuria and suprapubic pain
- **Setting:** Family Medicine Clinic

## PATIENT'S SIMULATED SCRIPT:

### Opening Statement:

"I've been feeling some burning when I pee, and I have this pain in my lower belly."

## HISTORY:

- **Pregnancy Details:**
  - G2P1, currently at 24 weeks' gestation.
  - First pregnancy was uneventful, normal vaginal delivery.
- **Symptoms:**
  - Burning sensation during urination (dysuria).
  - Suprapubic discomfort, described as a dull ache.
  - Increased frequency of urination without urgency.
  - No fever, flank pain, or vaginal discharge.

## PAST MEDICAL HISTORY:

- No known chronic conditions.
- No previous UTIs in pregnancy.

## DRUG HISTORY:

- **Regular Medications:** Folic acid 400 mcg daily, ferrous sulphate 325 mg daily.
- **Allergies:** No known drug allergies.

## OBSTETRIC HISTORY:

- Regular antenatal check-ups.
- No complications noted in the current pregnancy until now.

## FAMILY HISTORY:

- Mother has type 2 diabetes.
- Sister had preterm labour in her first pregnancy.

## LIFESTYLE AND SOCIAL HISTORY:

- Non-smoker, no alcohol consumption.
- Balanced diet, though admits to not drinking enough water daily.

## IDEAS, CONCERNS, EXPECTATIONS:

- **Ideas:** Thinks she may have diabetes because she has heard people feel like this and pass lots of urine when you are diabetic.
- **Concerns:** Worries this could harm her baby or lead to complications.
- **Expectations:** Hopes for a treatment plan that's safe for her pregnancy and effective.

## ON EXAMINATION:

- **General Appearance:** Appears well, no distress.
- **Vitals:** BP 112/70 mmHg, HR: 84 bpm, regular, temperature 36.8°C, $SpO_2$: 99% on room air.
- **Abdominal Examination:**
  - Uterus consistent with 24 weeks' gestation.
  - No uterine tenderness.
  - Suprapubic tenderness noted on palpation.
- **Urine Dipstick:**
  - Positive for nitrites and leukocytes.

## INVESTIGATIONS AND RESULTS:

1. **Urinalysis and Culture:**
   - Positive for *E. coli* (>100,000 CFU/mL), sensitive to nitrofurantoin.
2. **Blood Work:**
   - Normal renal function tests.
   - Normal haemoglobin and haematocrit levels.

## WHAT IS THE DIAGNOSIS?

**Urinary Tract Infection.**

A urinary tract infection (UTI) is an infection in any part of the urinary system, including the bladder, urethra, kidneys, or ureters. Most UTIs are bladder infections (cystitis) and are caused by bacteria, usually *E. coli*, entering the urinary tract.

## HOW WOULD YOU MANAGE THIS PATIENT?

*Immediate Steps:*

1. **Antibiotic Treatment:**
   - Start fosfomycin (1 dose only), alternatively nitrofurantoin (not at term).
2. **Symptom Management:**
   - Encourage increased water intake to help flush bacteria.
   - Provide paracetamol for discomfort if needed.

*Follow-up Plan:*

- Repeat urine culture 1–2 weeks after completing antibiotics to ensure resolution.
- Monitor for recurrence of symptoms.

## WHAT COMPLICATIONS CAN THE UTI CAUSE IF NOT TREATED?

- **Maternal Complications:**
  - Pyelonephritis, which can lead to sepsis.
  - Preterm labour or premature rupture of membranes.
- **Foetal Complications:**
  - Low birth weight.
  - Increased risk of foetal distress or preterm birth.

### Name three antibiotics which are considered safe in pregnancy for UTI treatment, and which should be avoided?

**Safe:**

- **Nitrofurantoin** (avoid near term due to risk of haemolytic anaemia in G6PD deficiency)
- **Cephalexin/cefuroxime**
- **Amoxicillin-clavulanate**

**Avoid:**

- **Trimethoprim-sulfamethoxazole** in first trimester (teratogenic risk) and near term (risk of kernicterus)
- **Fluoroquinolones** (risk of cartilage damage)
- **Tetracyclines** (teeth and bone abnormalities)

### What physiological changes in pregnancy predispose women to UTIs?

- **Urinary stasis** due to progesterone-mediated ureteral smooth muscle relaxation.
- **Hydronephrosis** of pregnancy from mechanical compression by the enlarging uterus.
- **Glycosuria** in the urine provides a nutrient-rich environment for bacterial growth.
- **Immune modulation** reduces ability to clear infections efficiently.

### What are the common causative organisms of UTI in pregnancy?

- ***Escherichia coli*** – accounts for 70–90% of cases.
- ***Klebsiella pneumoniae***
- ***Proteus mirabilis***
- ***Enterococcus faecalis***

*E. coli* is the most prevalent infective organism due to colonisation of the vaginal/periurethral areas alongside urinary stasis in pregnancy.

CASE

# Endometritis 28

## Doctor's Notes

*Patient Details:*

- **Name:** Lina Ahmed
- **Age:** 32
- **Occupation:** Accountant
- **Presenting Complaint:** Suprapubic pain, fever, and feeling unwell
- **Setting:** Family Medicine Clinic

## PATIENT'S SIMULATED SCRIPT:

### Opening Statement:

"I've been feeling really unwell with a fever and pain in my lower belly."

## HISTORY:

- **Onset and Course:**
  - Symptoms started 3 days ago.
  - Gradual onset of suprapubic pain, now constant and throbbing.
  - Fever (up to 39°C) with chills and sweating.
  - Feeling generally unwell and fatigued.
- **Associated Symptoms:**
  - Foul-smelling vaginal discharge.
  - Pain worsens with movement.
  - No urinary frequency or burning.
  - No nausea or vomiting.

## PAST MEDICAL HISTORY:

- Recent caesarean section 10 days ago due to foetal distress.
- No complications reported during surgery or immediate postpartum period.

## DRUG HISTORY:

- Paracetamol taken for fever and pain, with partial relief.
- Allergic to penicillin (reaction: rash and shortness of breath).

## OBSTETRIC HISTORY:

- G2P2, second pregnancy delivered via caesarean section.
- First pregnancy was a normal vaginal delivery with no complications.

## FAMILY HISTORY:

- No history of thromboembolic disorders or chronic illnesses in the family.

## LIFESTYLE AND SOCIAL HISTORY:

- Non-smoker, no alcohol consumption.
- Breastfeeding exclusively.

## IDEAS, CONCERNS, EXPECTATIONS:

- **Ideas:** Thinks it's her IBS flaring up.
- **Concerns:** Worries about an infection and whether it could affect her ability to care for her baby.
- **Expectations:** Hopes for treatment to relieve her symptoms and ensure no complications.

## ON EXAMINATION:

- **General Appearance:** Appears pale and unwell.
- **Vitals:** BP 110/70 mmHg, HR 110 bpm, regular, temperature 39°C, $SpO_2$: 97% on room air.
- **Abdominal Examination:**
  - Suprapubic tenderness, with guarding.
  - No rebound tenderness or palpable masses.
  - Uterus feels enlarged and tender on palpation.
- **Speculum Examination:**
  - Foul-smelling vaginal discharge.
  - No visible retained products of conception.
- **Pelvic Examination:**
  - Cervical motion tenderness.

## INVESTIGATIONS AND RESULTS:

1. **Blood Tests:**
   - **WBC:** 15,000/μL (elevated, neutrophil predominant).
   - **CRP:** 120 mg/L (elevated).
   - **Haemoglobin:** 10.8 g/dL (mild anaemia).
2. **Pelvic Ultrasound:**
   - Enlarged uterus with thickened endometrium (15 mm).
   - No retained products of conception or abscess.

## WHAT IS THE DIAGNOSIS?

**Postpartum Endometritis** (secondary to caesarean section).

Postpartum endometritis is an infection of the lining of the uterus (endometrium) that may occur after childbirth. It usually occurs when bacteria enter the uterus during delivery, especially after a caesarean section, prolonged labour, or when the water breaks too early.

## HOW WOULD YOU MANAGE THIS PATIENT?

*Immediate Steps:*

1. **Antibiotic Therapy:**
   - Start intravenous clindamycin 900 mg every 8 hours and gentamicin 5 mg/kg once daily (penicillin allergy – safe regimen).
   - Transition to oral antibiotics once afebrile and symptoms improve.
2. **Symptom Control:**
   - Continue paracetamol for fever and pain relief.
   - Encourage adequate hydration and rest.

*Follow-up Plan:*

- Monitor clinical improvement over 48 hours.
- If no improvement or worsening symptoms, consider further imaging to rule out abscess or retained products.

## WHAT ARE THE TYPICAL CLINICAL FEATURES OF POSTPARTUM ENDOMETRITIS?

The typical features include:

- Fever developing a few days (2–10) postpartum
- Foul smelling vaginal discharge or lochia.
- Cervical motion tenderness on bimanual examination
- Lower abdominal or suprapubic pain
- Tachycardia

### What are the major risk factors for postpartum endometritis?

- Caesarean section
- Prolonged labour/prolonged ruptured membranes
- Retained products of pregnancy
- Maternal comorbidities (diabetes, obesity or anaemia)

### What are potential complications of untreated postpartum endometritis?

- Sepsis/Shock
- Pelvic abscess formation
- Intrauterine adhesions or chronic endometritis
- Pelvic vein thrombosis

# CASE 29 Mastitis

## Doctor's Notes

*Patient Details:*

- **Name:** Sara Al-Ahmadi
- **Age:** 28
- **Occupation:** Homemaker
- **Presenting Complaint:** Painful and swollen left breast
- **Setting:** Family Medicine Clinic

## PATIENT'S SIMULATED SCRIPT

### Opening Statement:

"My left breast is painful, red, and swollen, and I feel feverish."

## HISTORY:

- **Onset and Course:**
  - Symptoms started 2 days ago with mild discomfort, which has worsened.
  - Redness and swelling noted yesterday.
  - Pain is localized to the upper outer quadrant of the left breast.
- **Associated Symptoms:**
  - Low-grade fever and feeling generally unwell.
  - No nipple discharge other than milk.
  - Breastfeeding difficulty due to pain on the affected side.

## PAST MEDICAL HISTORY:

- No previous episodes of mastitis.
- No history of breast surgeries or lumps.

## OBSTETRIC HISTORY:

- Delivered a healthy baby 4 months ago, normal vaginal delivery.

## DRUG HISTORY:

- Taking postnatal vitamins and iron supplements.
- No allergies.

## FAMILY HISTORY:

- No history of breast cancer or other breast conditions.

## LIFESTYLE AND SOCIAL HISTORY:

- Exclusively breastfeeding on demand.
- Well-supported by family, no significant stress.

## IDEAS, CONCERNS, EXPECTATIONS:

- **Ideas:** Thinks it might be because she's not making enough breastmilk.
- **Concerns:** Worries about whether she can continue breastfeeding or if the infection will affect her baby.
- **Expectations:** Hopes for a treatment to relieve the pain and swelling while continuing breastfeeding.

## ON EXAMINATION:

- **General Appearance:** Looks fatigued but not distressed.
- **Vitals:** BP 120/78 mmHg, HR90 bpm, regular, temperature 38.3°C (febrile).
- **Breast Examination:**
  - Left breast:
    - Redness and warmth over the upper outer quadrant.
    - Firm, tender swelling approximately 5 × 4 cm in size.
    - No fluctuation or obvious abscess formation.
    - No nipple cracks or visible fissures.
  - Right breast:
    - Normal, soft, non-tender.
- **Axillary Examination:**
  - Mildly enlarged, tender lymph nodes on the left side.

## INVESTIGATIONS:

1. **Clinical Diagnosis:** Typically sufficient for mastitis.
2. **Additional Investigations (if needed):**
   - Breast milk culture (if symptoms don't improve or if recurrent episodes occur).
   - Ultrasound if abscess suspected (none in this case).

## WHAT IS THE DIAGNOSIS?

**Lactational Mastitis** (infective).

Lactational mastitis is an infection of the breast tissue that can occur in breastfeeding women. It usually occurs when milk gets trapped in the breast and causes inflammation, creating an environment where bacteria can grow and cause an infection.

## HOW WOULD YOU MANAGE THIS PATIENT?

*Immediate Steps:*

1. **Symptom Relief:**
   - Paracetamol 500 mg every 6 hours or ibuprofen 400 mg every 8 hours for pain and fever.
2. **Antibiotic Therapy:**
   - Prescribe **cephalexin 500 mg** every 6 hours for 10 days.
   - If penicillin-allergic: Consider **clindamycin 300 mg** every 8 hours.
3. **Breastfeeding Support:**
   - Encourage continued breastfeeding from both breasts to prevent milk stasis.
   - Begin feedings on the unaffected side first to minimize pain.
   - Employ proper latching techniques to reduce recurrence.
   - Use a breast pump if pain prevents effective feeding.
4. **General Advice:**
   - Warm compresses before feeding to aid milk flow.
   - Cold compresses after feeding to reduce swelling and pain.
   - Adequate hydration and rest to support recovery.

## SAFETY NETTING:

- Advise to return or seek care if:
  - Fever persists or worsens after 48 hours of antibiotics.
  - An abscess develops (e.g., fluctuating swelling or worsening pain).
  - Symptoms recur after treatment.

## BENEFITS OF BREASTFEEDING:

1. **For the Baby:**
   - Provides ideal nutrition and is easily digestible.
   - Strengthens the immune system with antibodies, reducing infections.
   - Lowers risk of allergies, asthma, and obesity later in life.
2. **For the Mother:**
   - Promotes faster postpartum recovery and uterine contraction.
   - Lowers the risk of breast and ovarian cancer.
   - Improves bonding with the baby.
3. **For the Family:**
   - Economical and environmentally friendly.
   - Convenience of feeding without preparation.

## QUESTIONS:

1. **What are the common causes of mastitis?**
   - Milk stasis due to improper latching or infrequent feeding.
   - Nipple trauma or cracks, allowing bacterial entry.
2. **How can mastitis complications be prevented?**
   - Ensure proper breastfeeding techniques.
   - Early treatment to avoid abscess formation.
3. **How would you manage Mrs. Al-Ahmadi if she does not respond to oral antibiotics within 48–72 hours?**
   - Review the patient, order an ultrasound scan to check for abscess, consider IV antibiotics (if systemic symptoms)

4. **How would you manage recurrent mastitis in a breastfeeding mother?**
   - Reassess breastfeeding technique, check for nipple trauma or infant oral anomalies, encourage effective emptying of the breast, consider culture-directed antibiotics, and rarely use prophylaxis if recurrent.
5. **What is the rationale for prescribing cephalexin as first-line therapy in lactational mastitis?**
   - Covers common pathogens (*Staphylococcus aureus*, MSSA), is safe in breastfeeding, and has good tissue penetration with minimal side effects.

CASE 30

# Contraception Counselling

## Doctor's Notes

*Patient Details:*

- **Name:** Sarah A.
- **Age:** 32 years
- **Occupation:** Schoolteacher
- **Presenting Complaint:** Seeking contraception advice; specifically interested in the oral contraceptive pill
- **Setting:** Family Medicine Clinic

## PATIENT'S SIMULATED SCRIPT:

### Opening Statement:

"I've been using contraceptives for years, but I'm interested in switching to the oral contraceptive pill. I have high blood pressure and have been overweight for a while, so I'm wondering if the pill is safe for me."

## HISTORY:

Sarah is a 32-year-old woman with a history of hypertension (diagnosed 2 years ago) and obesity (BMI of 34 kg/m$^2$). She is currently in a stable relationship and does not plan for pregnancy at the moment. Her periods are regular, and she has no significant menstrual abnormalities. She reports taking lisinopril 10 mg daily to control her blood pressure, but she has not had regular follow-up appointments with her doctor for blood pressure management.

She denies any history of stroke, deep vein thrombosis (DVT), or other cardiovascular diseases. She has no history of smoking or diabetes and does not take any other medications.

## DRUG HISTORY:

- Lisinopril 10 mg daily for hypertension.
- No other current medications.

## FAMILY HISTORY:

- Mother: Hypertension and type 2 diabetes.
- Father: Healthy, no significant medical conditions.
- No family history of thromboembolic events.

## IDEAS, CONCERNS, EXPECTATIONS:

- **Ideas:** Sarah believes that the oral contraceptive pill would be a reliable and convenient method of contraception. She's heard about the pill previously and feels it may be the right option for her.
- **Concerns:** She is worried that you will say the pill might not be an option due to her general health and that she will have to get another method like a coil or contraceptive depot, which she is keen to avoid.
- **Expectations:** She expects to discuss safe contraceptive options that are suitable for her health conditions.

## ON EXAMINATION:

- **General Appearance:** Overweight, well-nourished.
- **Vital Signs:** BP 140/90 mmHg, pulse 82 bpm, respiratory rate 16/min, temperature 36.8°C.
- **Cardiovascular:** Regular rate and rhythm, no murmurs, no peripheral oedema.
- **Abdomen:** Soft, non-tender, no hepatosplenomegaly.
- **Extremities:** No signs of deep vein thrombosis, no varicosities.

## WHAT IS THE DIAGNOSIS?

- **Hypertension (uncontrolled).**
- **Obesity.**
- **Seeking contraception with a preference for the oral contraceptive pill.**

## HOW WOULD YOU ADVISE THIS PATIENT?

Given Sarah's medical history, it is important to avoid combined oral contraceptive pills (COCs) due to her hypertension and obesity, as the oestrogen component increases the risk of cardiovascular events.

*Recommended Contraceptive Options:*
- **Progestin-Only Pill (POP):** Safe for patients with hypertension and obesity, but requires strict adherence.
- **Intrauterine Device (IUD):** Either hormonal IUD or copper IUD. The hormonal IUD provides long-term contraception with minimal systemic side effects, and the copper IUD has no hormonal component, thus avoiding the risks of oestrogen.
- **Subdermal Implant:** A highly effective, long-acting reversible contraceptive option that contains progestin.
- **Contraceptive Injection:** Depo-Provera is an option, but weight gain is a possible side effect, which may not be ideal for Sarah given her obesity.

*Hypertension Management:*
- Sarah's blood pressure needs better control. Consider increasing her lisinopril dose or adding a calcium channel blocker or a thiazide diuretic for better management.

*Weight Management:*
- Referral to a dietitian for weight loss advice and exercise recommendations.
- Consider support for behavioural therapy if necessary, to assist with weight loss.

**What ethical considerations should be addressed in contraceptive counselling for Sarah?**

- Respect patient autonomy and preferences, provide full information on risks and benefits, balance maternal health and safety, ensure informed consent, and avoid coercion in contraceptive choice.

- Be aware that in the Middle East, in particular with Arab patients, the notion of contraception is associated with illicit behaviour (premarital intercourse), which is frowned upon, and non-evidence-based associations, e.g., that using the pill/contraception causes reduced fertility.

## FOLLOW-UP:

- Three-month follow-up to reassess blood pressure control, discuss contraception, and monitor for any side effects from the contraceptive method chosen.
- Regular monitoring of weight and lifestyle modifications to assist in obesity management.
- Schedule follow-up with a dietitian for dietary management and cardiovascular screening.

HRT

# CASE 31

## Doctor's Notes

*Patient Details:*

- **Name:** Laila M.
- **Age:** 55 years
- **Occupation:** Office Manager
- **Presenting Complaint:** Seeking advice on whether hormone replacement therapy (HRT) is suitable for her symptoms of hot flashes and low mood
- **Setting:** Family Medicine Clinic

## PATIENT'S SIMULATED SCRIPT:

### Opening Statement:

"I've been experiencing hot flashes and feel generally low lately. I've heard that hormone replacement therapy can help with these symptoms, and I wanted to know if it's a good option for me, considering my age and family history."

## HISTORY:

Laila is a 55-year-old woman who presents with complaints of hot flashes and low mood, which have been persistent for the past year. She reports that the symptoms are particularly bothersome during the night, disrupting her sleep. She also notes occasional irritability and fatigue, affecting her daily functioning. Laila has been postmenopausal for 3 years, with the cessation of her periods at age 52.

Her medical history is otherwise unremarkable, with no chronic illnesses such as diabetes, hypertension, or cardiovascular disease. She is not on any regular medications, except for occasional paracetamol for headache relief.

Laila has a family history of breast cancer (her mother was diagnosed at age 60), and she is concerned about the risks associated with HRT, especially due to this history.

## DRUG HISTORY:

- **Occasional paracetamol** (for headache relief).
- No regular medications.

## FAMILY HISTORY:

- **Mother**: Breast cancer, diagnosed at age 60 (currently in remission).
- **Father:** Hypertension, deceased at age 70 from a stroke.
- No family history of thromboembolic disease or cardiovascular disease.

## IDEAS, CONCERNS, EXPECTATIONS:

- **Ideas:** Laila believes that HRT could help alleviate her symptoms of hot flashes and low mood, improving her quality of life during menopause.
- **Concerns:** She is particularly worried about the potential breast cancer risk associated with HRT due to her family history. She is also concerned about possible side effects, such as weight gain, blood clots, or cardiovascular problems.
- **Expectations:** Laila hopes to receive guidance on whether HRT is suitable for her, given her family history and symptoms, and to understand the potential risks and benefits of treatment.

## ON EXAMINATION:

- **General Appearance**: Well-nourished, no signs of distress.
- **Vital Signs**: BP 120/80 mmHg, pulse 78 bpm, respiratory rate 16/min, temperature 36.6°C.
- **Cardiovascular**: Regular rate and rhythm, no murmurs.
- **Abdomen**: Soft, non-tender, no hepatosplenomegaly.
- **Breast Examination**: No lumps, no skin changes or axillary swelling.
- **Pelvic Examination**: No abnormalities.
- **Other Systems**: Unremarkable.

## WHAT IS THE DIAGNOSIS?

- **Menopausal Symptoms** (hot flashes, low mood).
- **Postmenopausal Status** (since age 52).
- **Family History of Breast Cancer.**

Menopause is a natural stage in a woman's life when her periods stop permanently, marking the end of her reproductive years. It usually happens between the ages of 45 and 55, but it can occur earlier or later.

Menopause occurs because the ovaries stop releasing eggs and produce lower levels of hormones like oestrogen and progesterone. These hormones regulate menstrual periods and help with functions like bone health, mood, and metabolism.

## HOW WOULD YOU MANAGE THIS PATIENT?

Given Laila's menopausal symptoms and her family history of breast cancer, the risks and benefits of HRT need to be carefully weighed.

HRT is generally effective in managing hot flashes, mood disturbances, and other symptoms of menopause, but it may have risks, especially in women with a family history of breast cancer.

### Options:

1. **Non-hormonal treatment options:**
    - **Selective serotonin reuptake inhibitors (SSRIs)** or **serotonin–norepinephrine reuptake inhibitors (SNRIs):** These medications can help manage mood symptoms like low mood and irritability and may also help with hot flashes.

- **Gabapentin**: Useful for hot flashes, especially during the night.
- **Clonidine**: A medication primarily used for hypertension but can also reduce hot flashes.
- **Lifestyle modifications:** Including regular exercise, a balanced diet, and sleep hygiene may also help improve her symptoms.

2. **HRT:**
   - **Oestrogen-only HRT:** This may be appropriate for women who have had a **hysterectomy**. However, Laila still has her uterus, so oestrogen alone would not be suitable.
   - **Combined oestrogen and progesterone therapy:** This could relieve hot flashes and mood symptoms. However, due to Laila's **family history of breast cancer,** there are concerns about potential **increased breast cancer risk** with long-term use of combined HRT.
   - **Bioidentical hormone therapy** or **local oestrogen therapy:** Given her family history of breast cancer, **bioidentical hormone therapy** or **local oestrogen therapy (e.g., vaginal creams or rings)** could be considered, though they are less effective for hot flashes compared to systemic HRT.
3. **Breast cancer screening:**
   - **Annual mammogram:** Since her family history of breast cancer places her at higher risk, it is important to continue regular mammogram screenings. Her last mammogram was negative.
   - **Referral to a genetic counsellor:** If her family history of breast cancer is significant, discussing her **genetic risk** for breast cancer may provide more tailored guidance regarding HRT.

### What screening should be done before initiating HRT in a woman with a family history of breast cancer?

- Ensure up-to-date mammogram, consider referral to genetic counselling if family history is significant, assess personal risk factors (age, BMI).

### How can family physicians integrate patient preferences in menopausal symptom management?

- Provide shared decision-making, educate on risks and benefits, respect patient choice for therapy type, tailor interventions to symptom severity, comorbidities, and lifestyle.

### How could local or bioidentical HRT be used for Laila?

- Local vaginal oestrogen can relieve urogenital symptoms with minimal systemic absorption. Bioidentical hormones may be considered, but evidence is limited; systemic symptom control is less effective than standard HRT.

## FOLLOW-UP:

- Follow-up in 2 months to assess the effectiveness of non-hormonal treatments or any changes in her symptoms if she chooses a pharmacological approach.
- Regular mammograms as per guidelines (annually) due to her family history.
- Consider genetic counselling to evaluate her personal risk of breast cancer.
- Reassess mood and hot flashes to determine if further intervention is needed.

## SAFETY NETTING:

- Advise Laila to seek medical attention if she experiences any breast lumps, unusual pain, or changes in her breasts, as well as any new vaginal bleeding or other symptoms that could indicate side effects from HRT or other treatments.
- If she experiences severe headaches, chest pain, or signs of deep vein thrombosis (e.g., swelling or pain in the legs), she should seek immediate medical help.

CASE 32

# Antiphospholipid Syndrome

## Doctor's Notes

*Patient Details:*

- **Name:** Noor S.
- **Age:** 28 years
- **Occupation:** Office assistant
- **Presenting Complaint:** Seeking advice about recurrent miscarriages and management of recently diagnosed antiphospholipid syndrome (APS)
- **Setting:** Family Medicine Clinic

## PATIENT'S SIMULATED SCRIPT:

### Opening Statement:

"I've had three miscarriages in the past, and my doctor recently told me I have antiphospholipid syndrome. I'm on the pill right now, but I want to understand what I should do to manage my condition and plan for the future."

## HISTORY:

Noor is a 28-year-old woman who presents with a history of three first-trimester miscarriages, the last occurring a year ago. After a series of tests, she was diagnosed with antiphospholipid syndrome (APS), confirmed by persistently positive antiphospholipid antibodies on two separate occasions at least 12 weeks apart.

She is currently on the oral contraceptive pill (combined) for contraception, which she started after her last miscarriage. Noor reports no history of venous or arterial thromboembolic events (e.g., deep vein thrombosis [DVT], stroke). She is otherwise healthy, with no significant comorbidities.

She does not smoke or drink alcohol. She expresses a strong desire to have children in the future and wants to know how her APS can be managed to improve her chances of a successful pregnancy.

## DRUG HISTORY:

- Combined oral contraceptive (COC) pill for contraception.
- No other regular medications.

## FAMILY HISTORY:

- **Mother:** Hypertension, no history of thrombosis or autoimmune disease.
- **Father:** Type 2 diabetes.
- **No family history** of recurrent miscarriages, thromboembolic events, or autoimmune conditions.

## IDEAS, CONCERNS, EXPECTATIONS:

- **Ideas:** Noor wonders if she is just genetically predisposed to having miscarriages. She saw once on a television show that a character had a harsh environment in her womb and as a result could not carry a child to term.
- **Concerns:** She is worried about her ability to have a successful pregnancy in the future. Additionally, she's concerned about the safety of continuing the oral contraceptive pill, given her diagnosis of APS.
- **Expectations:** She expects clear guidance on managing APS, especially in the context of pregnancy planning. She also wants advice on safe contraception in the meantime.

## ON EXAMINATION:

- **General Appearance**: Healthy-looking, no signs of acute illness.
- **Vital Signs**: BP 118/76 mmHg, pulse 80 bpm, respiratory rate 16/min, temperature 36.7°C.
- **Cardiovascular**: Normal heart sounds, no murmurs, no peripheral oedema.
- **Respiratory**: Clear lung fields, no abnormalities.
- **Extremities**: No signs of DVT (no swelling, erythema, or tenderness).
- **Other Systems**: Unremarkable.

## WHAT IS THE DIAGNOSIS?

- **Antiphospholipid Syndrome (APS)** – Confirmed diagnosis with a history of recurrent miscarriages.
- Current use of combined oral contraceptive pill (not ideal for patients with APS).

APS is a condition where the immune system mistakenly creates antibodies that increase the risk of blood clots. These abnormal clots can form in the veins or arteries, leading to serious complications such as DVT, stroke, or pregnancy complications.

## HOW WOULD YOU MANAGE THIS PATIENT?

1. **Management of APS:**
   - **Pre-pregnancy planning:**
     - Discontinue the COC immediately, as it increases the risk of thrombosis in APS.
     - Offer alternative contraception methods:
       - Progestin-only pill, intrauterine device (IUD) (hormonal or copper), or barrier methods.
     - Advise Noor to wait until APS is adequately managed and a thorough pre-pregnancy plan is in place before attempting to conceive.
   - **During pregnancy:**
     - Start **low-dose aspirin (75–150 mg daily)** and **low-molecular-weight heparin (LMWH)** as soon as pregnancy is confirmed. These are the standard treatments to reduce the risk of pregnancy complications in APS.
     - Ensure close monitoring during pregnancy by a multidisciplinary team, including a maternal–fetal medicine specialist, haematologist, and obstetrician.
   - **For thrombotic risk management (non-pregnant state):**
     - If Noor has no history of thrombotic events, long-term anticoagulation may not be needed. Lifestyle modifications (e.g., avoiding smoking, maintaining a healthy weight, staying active) are essential.
     - Regular follow-up with her physician is needed to monitor her condition.

2. **Patient education:**
   - Educate Noor about the risks associated with APS, including pregnancy complications (e.g., preeclampsia, intrauterine growth restriction, or preterm birth) and potential thrombotic events.
   - Provide clear instructions on recognizing signs of thrombosis (e.g., leg pain/swelling, chest pain, shortness of breath) and seeking immediate medical care if they occur.

## SAFETY NETTING:

- Advise Noor to report any symptoms of thrombosis (e.g., leg swelling or pain, chest pain, or shortness of breath) immediately.
- Educate her on the importance of adherence to LMWH and aspirin therapy during pregnancy and the risks of stopping these treatments prematurely.
- Emphasize the need for regular health checks, including blood pressure monitoring and routine screenings, to reduce the risk of complications.

## HOW WOULD YOU MANAGE ANTIPHOSPHOLIPID SYNDROME (APS)?

- **Non-pregnant state:**
  - Avoid combined oral contraceptives due to thrombosis risk.
  - Lifestyle modifications to minimize thrombotic risk.
  - Long-term anticoagulation (e.g., warfarin or direct oral anticoagulants) may be required if there is a history of thrombosis.
- **During pregnancy:**
  - Start low-dose aspirin and LMWH at the earliest sign of pregnancy to reduce the risk of miscarriage and other complications.
  - Provide regular antenatal care and multidisciplinary monitoring.

### Why is the COC contraindicated in Noor?

- COCs increase the risk of thromboembolic events, which is already elevated in patients with APS. They should be discontinued immediately in this context.

### How should recurrent miscarriages be addressed in APS?

- Preconception planning with aspirin and LMWH prophylaxis, early confirmation of pregnancy, close monitoring, and counselling regarding the prognosis of successful pregnancy with therapy.

### When is long-term anticoagulation indicated in APS?

- In patients with a history of venous or arterial thrombosis, lifelong anticoagulation (e.g., warfarin) is indicated. In asymptomatic patients with obstetric APS only, long-term anticoagulation is not required.

CASE 33

# Molar Pregnancy

## Doctor's Notes

*Patient Details:*

- **Name:** Sarah A.
- **Age:** 32 years
- **Occupation:** Teacher
- **Presenting Complaint:** Nausea, vomiting, and vaginal bleeding during early pregnancy.
- **Setting:** Family Medicine Clinic, referred for evaluation after symptoms began 2 days ago.

## PATIENT'S SIMULATED SCRIPT:

### Opening Statement:

"I've been feeling extremely nauseous, and I've had some bleeding for the past 2 days. I don't feel well, and I'm worried about my pregnancy."

## HISTORY:

Sarah is a 32-year-old pregnant woman, approximately 9 weeks' gestation by her last menstrual period (LMP). She presents with severe nausea and vomiting, which have significantly worsened over the past week. She has also experienced intermittent vaginal bleeding, described as light to moderate, over the past 2 days.

She denies any abdominal pain or cramping but reports dizziness and feeling lightheaded, particularly when standing up. She feels weaker than usual and is unable to keep down solid food or liquids.

Sarah has no prior history of miscarriage or complications in previous pregnancies. This is her second pregnancy, and her first pregnancy was uneventful.

She has no significant past medical history, takes no regular medications, and denies smoking or alcohol use.

## DRUG HISTORY:

- No regular medications.
- Occasionally uses paracetamol for headaches.

## FAMILY HISTORY:

- No history of molar pregnancies, miscarriages, or genetic conditions.
- Both parents are alive and well with no major medical concerns.

## IDEAS, CONCERNS, EXPECTATIONS:

- **Ideas:** Sarah believes her symptoms might be related to her pregnancy but is unsure why her nausea and vomiting are so severe.
- **Concerns:** She is worried about the cause of her bleeding and whether it means she might lose the pregnancy. She is also concerned about her overall health, particularly her dizziness and inability to eat or drink.
- **Expectations:** Sarah expects an explanation for her symptoms and immediate management of her condition. She is hoping to understand whether her pregnancy is viable and what steps need to be taken next.

## ON EXAMINATION:

- **General Appearance:** Pale, appears weak, moderately distressed.
- **Vital Signs:** BP 92/58 mmHg (slightly hypotensive), pulse 102 bpm (tachycardic), temperature 36.8°C, respiratory rate 18/min.
- **Abdominal Examination:**
  - Abdomen soft, non-tender, no palpable masses.
  - No guarding or rebound tenderness.
- **Pelvic Examination:**
  - Vaginal bleeding noted, no active heavy bleeding at the time of examination.
  - No cervical motion tenderness or adnexal masses.

## ULTRASOUND FINDINGS:

- Ultrasound shows a heterogeneous intrauterine mass with multiple anechoic spaces resembling a "snowstorm" appearance, consistent with a molar pregnancy.
- No foetal pole or cardiac activity is detected.

## WHAT IS THE DIAGNOSIS?

**Molar Pregnancy** (hydatidiform mole) with symptoms of hyperemesis gravidarum, vaginal bleeding, and possible hypovolemia.

A molar pregnancy is a rare complication where a pregnancy starts abnormally. Instead of a healthy baby developing, there is an abnormal growth of tissue in the uterus due to a problem with fertilization. This tissue, called a mole, can grow uncontrollably and sometimes even turn cancerous if not treated.

### What immediate management steps are needed for Sarah?

- Stabilize hydration and electrolytes with IV fluids, correct hypotension and electrolyte imbalances, administer anti-emetics, monitor vital signs, and promptly refer to obstetrics and gynaecology.

### What is the definitive treatment for a molar pregnancy?

- Uterine evacuation via suction curettage, with histopathological confirmation of molar tissue. Ensure blood products are available in case of significant bleeding.

### How should Sarah be monitored after molar pregnancy evacuation?

- Serial β-hCG measurements weekly until undetectable, then monthly for 6–12 months to detect persistent trophoblastic disease or gestational trophoblastic neoplasia.

**What contraception advice should be given after a molar pregnancy?**

- Advise against pregnancy for 6–12 months until β-hCG levels normalize; recommend reliable contraception such as a progestin-only method or IUD.

**What are the potential complications of molar pregnancy that need monitoring?**

- Heavy bleeding, infection, persistent gestational trophoblastic disease, invasive mole, or choriocarcinoma. Prompt recognition and follow-up are critical.

CASE 34

# Cervical Insufficiency

## Doctor's Notes

*Patient Details:*

- **Name:** Fatima Al-Hassan
- **Age:** 28
- **Occupation:** Teacher
- **Presenting Complaint:** First antenatal visit
- **Setting:** Family Medicine Clinic

## PATIENT'S SIMULATED SCRIPT:

### Opening Statement:

"I'm here for my first pregnancy check-up."

## HISTORY:

- **Obstetric History:**
  - Gravida 2 Para 0 (G2P0).
  - Previous miscarriage at 14 weeks; required anti-D injection at that time.
  - No previous live births or ectopic pregnancies.
- **Current Pregnancy History:**
  - Positive home pregnancy test 7 weeks ago.
  - No bleeding or abdominal pain.
  - No nausea, vomiting, or urinary complaints.

## PAST MEDICAL HISTORY:

- Previous miscarriage.
- No history of hypertension, diabetes, or thyroid disorders.

## DRUG HISTORY:

- Folic acid 400 mcg daily.
- No other medications.
- No known drug allergies.

## FAMILY HISTORY:

- Mother has hypertension.
- No family history of congenital anomalies or recurrent miscarriages.

## LIFESTYLE AND SOCIAL HISTORY:

- Non-smoker, no alcohol use.
- Balanced diet but admits to skipping meals due to her busy teaching schedule.
- Lives with supportive husband.

## IDEAS, CONCERNS, EXPECTATIONS:

- **Ideas:** Wants to confirm that the pregnancy is progressing normally.
- **Concerns:** Afraid of miscarrying again.
- **Expectations:** Hoping for reassurance and guidance to avoid complications.

## ON EXAMINATION:

- **General Appearance:** Well and comfortable.
- **Vital Signs:** BP 110/70 mmHg, HR 82 bpm, regular, temperature 36.8°C.
- **Abdominal Examination:**
  - Abdomen soft, non-tender.
  - Fundal height consistent with gestational age.
- **Pelvic Examination:**
  - Cervix dilated to 1.5 cm.
  - No active bleeding or discharge.

## INVESTIGATIONS:

1. **Blood Tests:**
   - **Blood Group:** Rh-negative.
   - **Husband's Blood Group:** Rh-positive.
   - **Haemoglobin:** 12.4 g/dL.
   - **Renal:** Normal glucose and renal function tests.
2. **Ultrasound:**
   - Viable intrauterine pregnancy at 9 weeks' gestation.
   - Normal foetal heart activity.
   - No signs of retrochorionic haemorrhage or placental issues.

## WHAT IS THE DIAGNOSIS?

1. **Cervical Insufficiency** with early dilation.
2. **Rh Incompatibility Risk** (Rh-negative mother and Rh-positive father).

Cervical insufficiency (also called incompetent cervix) is when the cervix weakens and opens too early during pregnancy, before the baby is ready to be born. This can lead to miscarriage or preterm birth (early delivery), usually in the second trimester (weeks 14–27).

## MANAGEMENT PLAN:

*Immediate Steps:*

1. **Cervical Insufficiency:**
   - Refer urgently to obstetrics for cervical cerclage.
   - Advise bed rest and avoidance of heavy lifting or strenuous activity until cerclage is performed.
   - Monitor for signs of infection, contractions, or vaginal bleeding.
2. **Rh Incompatibility:**
   - Administer anti-D immunoglobulin to prevent Rh sensitization.
   - Schedule routine anti-D administration at 28 weeks and after delivery if the baby is Rh-positive.
3. **General Antenatal Care:**
   - Continue folic acid 400 mcg daily.
   - Advise on balanced nutrition, adequate hydration, and iron-rich foods.
   - Regular antenatal visits to monitor foetal growth and maternal health.

*Long-Term Management:*

- Plan regular ultrasounds to monitor cervical length.
- Educate about recognizing symptoms of preterm labour or miscarriage.

## QUESTIONS:

1. **When do you perform a cervical cerclage?**
   - Typically done at 12–14 weeks' gestation for cervical insufficiency.
2. **What are the complications of cervical cerclage?**
   - Infection, preterm labour, rupture of membranes, or cervical trauma.
3. **How do you manage Rh incompatibility?**
   - Administer anti-D immunoglobulin at 28 weeks' gestation and postpartum if the baby is Rh-positive.
   - Additional doses are needed after any event that might cause geomaterial haemorrhage (e.g., miscarriage, trauma, or procedures such as amniocentesis).
4. **What is the relevance of Rh incompatibility in this patient?**
   - Mother is Rh-negative, father is Rh-positive; risk of haemolytic disease of the foetus and newborn if maternal sensitization occurs.
5. **How is cervical length monitored during pregnancy?**
   - Transvaginal ultrasounds to measure cervical length; a shortening cervix may indicate risk of preterm birth and need for early intervention.

# CASE 35
# Antenatal Visit – Hypothyroidism

## Doctor's Notes

*Patient Details:*

- **Name:** Laila Ahmad
- **Age:** 30
- **Occupation:** Office assistant
- **Presenting Complaint:** First antenatal visit and neck swelling
- **Setting:** Family Medicine Clinic

## PATIENT'S SIMULATED SCRIPT:

### Opening Statement:

"I'm here for my first pregnancy checkup, but I've also noticed a lump in my neck."

## HISTORY:

- **Obstetric History:**
  - Gravida 2 Para 1 (G2P1).
  - Previous pregnancy uneventful, normal vaginal delivery at term.
  - No history of miscarriage or pregnancy complications.
- **Current Pregnancy History:**
  - Positive home pregnancy test 8 weeks ago.
  - No nausea, vomiting, or abdominal pain.
  - No bleeding or spotting.
- **Neck Swelling History:**
  - Swelling noticed 2 months ago, has not changed significantly in size.
  - No pain, redness, or tenderness.
  - No history of dysphagia, dyspnoea, or hoarseness.

- **Associated Symptoms:**
  - Mild fatigue, constipation, and dry skin for several months.
  - No heat or cold intolerance.
  - No family history of thyroid issues or malignancies.

## PAST MEDICAL HISTORY:

- No known chronic conditions.

## DRUG HISTORY:

- Folic acid 400 mcg daily.
- No other medications.
- No known drug allergies.

## FAMILY HISTORY:

- Mother has hypothyroidism.
- Father has hypertension.

## LIFESTYLE AND SOCIAL HISTORY:

- Non-smoker, no alcohol use.
- Balanced diet.
- Lives with supportive husband and one child.

## IDEAS, CONCERNS, EXPECTATIONS:

- **Ideas:** Wonders if the lump in her neck is dangerous.
- **Concerns:** Fears it could be cancer.
- **Expectations:** Hopes for a clear diagnosis and reassurance.

## ON EXAMINATION:

- **General Appearance:** Well and alert.
- **Vital Signs:** BP 110/70 mmHg, HR 80 bpm, regular, temperature 36.6°C.
- **Neck Examination:**
  - 4 cm × 4 cm nodule in the right thyroid lobe, non-tender, firm, and mobile.
  - No overlying skin changes or palpable cervical lymphadenopathy.
- **Abdominal Examination:**
  - Uterus consistent with 8 weeks' gestation.
- **Systemic Examination:** Normal findings.

## INVESTIGATIONS:

1. **Blood Tests:**
   - **TSH:** 13 mIU/L (elevated, hypothyroid).
   - **Free T4:** Low (exact value to be provided if asked).
   - Normal CBC and renal function.

2. **Neck Ultrasound:**
   - Single 4 cm × 4 cm thyroid nodule in the right lobe.
   - No suspicious features or vascularity.
3. **Fine Needle Aspiration (FNA):**
   - Bethesda 2 classification: Benign cytology.

## WHAT IS THE DIAGNOSIS?

1. **Subclinical or Overt Hypothyroidism** secondary to thyroid nodule.
2. **Benign Thyroid Nodule (Bethesda 2).**

Hypothyroidism in pregnancy occurs when the thyroid gland (a small butterfly-shaped gland in the neck) doesn't make enough thyroid hormones, which are essential for the baby's brain development and the body's metabolism.

The most common cause is Hashimoto's thyroiditis, an autoimmune condition where the body mistakenly attacks the thyroid. Other causes include iodine deficiency, previous thyroid surgery, or certain medications.

## HOW WOULD YOU MANAGE THIS PATIENT?

*Immediate Steps:*

1. **Thyroid Nodule:**
   - Reassure the patient that the nodule is benign (Bethesda 2).
   - Regular ultrasound monitoring of the nodule every 6–12 months.
2. **Hypothyroidism:**
   - Initiate levothyroxine therapy at a pregnancy-adjusted dose (e.g., 50–75 mcg daily) to normalize TSH.
   - Target TSH level in the first trimester: <2.5 mIU/L.
   - Monitor TSH levels every 4–6 weeks during pregnancy to adjust the dose as needed.
3. **Antenatal Care:**
   - Continue folic acid 400 mcg daily.
   - Routine antenatal blood work and booking ultrasound at 12 weeks.
   - Provide dietary advice to ensure iodine adequacy (e.g., iodized salt, dairy products, and fish).

*Long-Term Management:*

- Postpartum thyroid function test to reassess levothyroxine needs.
- Continued monitoring of thyroid nodule size and function.

## SAFETY NETTING:

- Seek urgent care if:
  - Swelling becomes painful or rapidly enlarges.
  - Difficulty breathing or swallowing develops.

## QUESTIONS:

1. **What is the Bethesda classification system?**
   - A system used to classify thyroid FNA cytology results into six categories, each with specific management recommendations. Bethesda 2 indicates a benign nodule with a very low risk of malignancy.
2. **Why is hypothyroidism important to treat in pregnancy?**
   - Untreated hypothyroidism can lead to complications such as miscarriage, preterm birth, low birth weight, and impaired foetal brain development.

3. **What is the target TSH level during pregnancy?**
   - First trimester: <2.5 mIU/L.
   - Second and third trimesters: <3.0 mIU/L.
4. **What complications can occur if hypothyroidism is untreated later in pregnancy?**
   - Maternal complications: anemia, preeclampsia, placental abruption.
   - Foetal complications: neurodevelopmental delay, low IQ, and growth restriction.

CASE

# Premarital Counselling 36

## Doctor's Notes

*Patient Details:*

- **Name:** Ahmed Al-Sayed
- **Age:** 27
- **Occupation:** Engineer
- **Presenting Complaint:** Premarital counselling
- **Setting:** Family Medicine Clinic

## PATIENT'S SIMULATED SCRIPT:

### Opening Statement:

"I'm here because I need the premarital tests and advice."

## ARAB BOARD EXPECTATIONS FOR RESIDENT DOCTOR:

- Address cultural sensitivities and expectations related to marriage.
- Perform a thorough medical history and examination.
- Provide evidence-based advice about genetic, infectious, and chronic disease screening.
- Discuss family planning, fertility, and lifestyle modifications to ensure a healthy marriage and potential pregnancy.

## HISTORY:

- **Personal History:**
  - No known chronic illnesses.
  - No surgical history.
  - No history of blood disorders or genetic diseases.
- **Family History:**
  - No family history of genetic disorders or chronic conditions such as diabetes or hypertension.

- **Lifestyle History:**
  - Non-smoker, no alcohol use.
  - Regular exercise: jogging 3 times a week.
  - Balanced diet with no specific restrictions.
- **Infectious Disease History:**
  - No history of tuberculosis, hepatitis, or sexually transmitted infections (STIs).
- **Reproductive Health History:**
  - No previous sexual relationships.
  - Aware of the importance of family planning but has limited knowledge of contraception.
- **Genetic History:**
  - His cousin has sickle cell disease, but there are no other known genetic disorders in the family.
- **Immunization History:**
  - Up to date on childhood vaccinations but unsure about hepatitis B vaccination.

## IDEAS, CONCERNS, EXPECTATIONS:

- **Ideas:** Wants to ensure he and his future spouse are compatible in terms of health.
- **Concerns:** Worried about the potential for genetic disorders given his cousin's condition.
- **Expectations:** Hopes to receive comprehensive guidance and clearance for marriage.

## ON EXAMINATION:

- **General Appearance:** Well and healthy-looking.
- **Vital Signs:** BP 120/76 mmHg, HR 72 bpm, regular, temperature 36.5°C.
- **Systemic Examination:** Normal findings.

## INVESTIGATIONS:

1. **Premarital Screening Tests:**
   - **Complete Blood Count (CBC):** Normal.
   - **Haemoglobin Electrophoresis:** Carrier of sickle cell trait (AS).
   - **Hepatitis B and C Screening:** Negative.
   - **HIV Test:** Negative.
   - **Rubella IgG:** Positive (immunity present).
   - **Syphilis (RPR):** Negative.

## WHAT IS THE DIAGNOSIS?

**Sickle Cell Trait (AS) Carrier.**

Sickle cell trait means the individual has inherited one normal blood cell gene and one sickle cell gene from their parents. It is not a disease, and most people with sickle cell trait do not have any health problems. However, in rare cases, extreme physical stress, dehydration, or high altitudes can cause complications. The main thing to know is that the sickle cell gene can be passed to one's children.

Sickle cell disease is a blood condition an individual is born with that affects how their red blood cells work. Normally, red blood cells are round and move easily through blood vessels, but in sickle cell disease, some red blood cells become hard, sticky, and are shaped like a crescent or sickle. These sickle-shaped cells can block blood flow, causing pain, organ damage, and other health problems.

## MANAGEMENT PLAN:

*Immediate Steps:*

1. **Genetic Counselling:**
   - If the future spouse is also a carrier of sickle cell trait or other haemoglobinopathies, counsel about the 25% risk of having a child with sickle cell disease.
   - Offer referral to a genetic counsellor if needed.
2. **Infectious Disease Prevention:**
   - Confirm hepatitis B vaccination status. If unvaccinated, initiate vaccination series.
3. **Health Optimization:**
   - Encourage maintaining a healthy lifestyle to reduce the risk of chronic diseases.
   - Provide preconception advice if planning for children, including folic acid supplementation.

*Lifestyle and Family Planning Advice:*

- Discuss the importance of a balanced diet, exercise, and stress management for marital and family health.
- Educate about available contraceptive methods and when to use them.
- If planning children, recommend preconception folic acid 400 mcg daily.

*Long-Term Recommendations:*

- Follow-up for hepatitis B vaccination.
- Ensure spouse also undergoes premarital screening.

## QUESTIONS:

1. **Why is premarital counselling important?**
   - To identify and address genetic, infectious, and chronic conditions that may impact the health of the couple or their future children.
2. **What should a carrier of sickle cell trait do before marriage?**
   - Ensure the partner is tested for sickle cell trait or disease and seek genetic counselling if both are carriers.
3. **What are the benefits of hepatitis B vaccination in this context?**
   - Prevents transmission of hepatitis B, a serious infection that can lead to chronic liver disease and cancer.
4. **Why is folic acid important for preconception care?**
   - Reduces the risk of neural tube defects in the developing foetus.
5. **What should a carrier of sickle cell trait do before marriage?**
   - Ensure the partner is tested for sickle cell trait or disease; seek genetic counselling if both are carriers to understand the 25% risk of having a child with sickle cell disease.

# CASE 37 Croup

## Doctor's Notes

*Patient Details:*

- **Name:** Omar Hassan
- **Age:** 3 years
- **Accompanied by:** Mother
- **Presenting Complaint:** Cough for 3 days
- **Setting:** Family Medicine Clinic

## PATIENT'S SIMULATED SCRIPT:

### Opening Statement:

"My son has had this strange cough for a few days. I even recorded it for you to hear."

## HISTORY:

- **Symptom Onset:**
  - Started 3 days ago with a mild fever and runny nose.
- **Cough Details:**
  - Barking cough, especially noticeable at night.
  - No wheezing or choking episodes.
  - Video shows a characteristic barking sound.
- **Associated Symptoms:**
  - Hoarseness of voice.
  - No difficulty swallowing; no drooling.
  - Mild difficulty breathing during the cough episodes.
- **Systemic Symptoms:**
  - Fever (up to 38.5°C).
  - Otherwise active and playful.

- **Past Medical History:**
  - No previous hospital admissions or serious illnesses.
  - No history of asthma or allergies.
- **Birth and Developmental History:**
  - Full-term normal delivery.
  - Milestones achieved appropriately.
- **Immunization History:**
  - Up to date with vaccinations.
- **Social History:**
  - Lives with parents and two older siblings who recently had cold symptoms.
  - Attends daycare.

## IDEAS, CONCERNS, EXPECTATIONS:

- **Ideas:** Mother suspects a viral infection due to recent cold symptoms in siblings.
- **Concerns:** Worried about the unusual sound of the cough and potential breathing difficulties.
- **Expectations:** Hopes for reassurance and a clear treatment plan.

## ON EXAMINATION:

- **General Appearance:** Child appears alert and well, mildly irritable during coughing episodes.
- **Vital Signs:** Temperature 37.8°C, HR 110 bpm, RR 24 breaths/min, $SpO_2$: 96% on room air.
- **Respiratory Examination:**
  - Stridor heard on inspiration, more prominent when agitated.
  - Chest clear with no wheezing or crackles.
  - No chest wall retractions.
- **ENT Examination:**
  - No drooling or tonsillar swelling.
  - Mild erythema of the throat.

## INVESTIGATIONS:

No additional investigations needed, as clinical presentation is consistent with croup.

## WHAT IS THE DIAGNOSIS?

**Croup (laryngotracheobronchitis).**

Croup is a common respiratory illness in young children that leads to swelling of the upper airways, resulting in a distinctive barking cough, hoarseness, and sometimes a high-pitched noise when breathing in, known as stridor. It is typically caused by viral infections, with the parainfluenza virus being a frequent culprit. Symptoms often start like a cold, with a runny nose and fever, and then progress to the characteristic cough and breathing difficulties.

## MANAGEMENT PLAN:

*Immediate Steps:*

1. **Supportive Care:**
   - Reassure the mother about the benign nature of croup in most cases.
   - Advise on maintaining hydration and using a cool-mist humidifier at home.

2. **Pharmacological Management:**
   - Prescribe a single dose of oral dexamethasone (0.15 mg/kg) to reduce inflammation and severity of symptoms.
   - Instruct the mother to monitor for signs of worsening (e.g., stridor at rest, increased work of breathing).
3. **Safety Netting:**
   - Advise seeking urgent care if:
     - Stridor occurs at rest or worsens.
     - Difficulty breathing or cyanosis develops.
     - The child becomes lethargic or stops drinking fluids.

*Follow-up:*
- Routine follow-up is not necessary if symptoms improve, but the mother is encouraged to call or return if concerned.

## PARENT EDUCATION:

- **What is Croup?**
  - A viral infection causing swelling of the voice box and windpipe, leading to the characteristic barking cough.
- **Home Care Tips:**
  - Keep the child calm to prevent worsening stridor.
  - Encourage fluids and ensure adequate rest.
  - Use steam inhalation sparingly, as cool air is often more effective.
- **Prognosis:**
  - Symptoms usually resolve in 3–7 days.

## CONSULTATION WRAP-UP:

- **"Do you feel more reassured about Omar's condition?"**
- **"Do you have any further questions or concerns about his care?"**

## QUESTIONS:

1. **What are the red flags in a child with croup?**
   - Stridor at rest, significant chest wall retractions, lethargy, or cyanosis.
2. **How does dexamethasone help in croup?**
   - Reduces airway inflammation, improving symptoms within 2–3 hours.
3. **What are the benefits of keeping the child calm during an episode?**
   - Reduces respiratory effort and prevents worsening of stridor.
4. **How do you classify the severity of croup?**
   - **Mild:** Barking cough, no stridor at rest, minimal/no retractions.
   - **Moderate:** Stridor at rest, mild–moderate retractions, minimal distress.
   - **Severe:** Prominent stridor at rest, severe retractions, agitation/lethargy, hypoxia.
   - **Impending respiratory failure:** Fatigue, decreased stridor (airflow reduced), cyanosis, altered mental state.
5. **Why should the child be kept calm during an episode?**
   - Agitation increases oxygen demand and worsens stridor due to increased turbulence in narrowed airways. Keeping the child calm reduces risk of airway compromise.

CASE 38

# Failure to Thrive

## Doctor's Notes

*Patient Details:*

- **Name:** Ahmad Ali
- **Age:** 8 months
- **Accompanied by:** Mother
- **Presenting Complaint:** Failure to gain weight, shortness of breath, and fatigue
- **Setting:** Family Medicine Clinic

## PATIENT'S SIMULATED SCRIPT:

### Opening Statement:

"My baby is very tired and doesn't seem to be growing like other children his age."

## HISTORY:

- **Growth and Development History:**
  - Birth weight was normal, but Ahmad has been steadily dropping on the growth chart in the last 3 months.
  - Weight now below the 5th percentile for his age.
  - Developmental milestones delayed, especially motor skills.
- **Current Symptoms:**
  - Persistent fatigue, tires easily during feeding.
  - Shortness of breath with mild exertion.
  - Pale skin and occasional irritability.
- **Dietary History:**
  - Exclusively breastfed for 6 months; started on solid foods, but intake is minimal.
  - No issues with breastfeeding initially.
- **Family History:**
  - Parents are first cousins.
  - One older sibling died at 2 years of age due to "severe anaemia."

- **Birth History:**
  - Full-term normal vaginal delivery.
  - No complications during pregnancy or delivery.
- **Social History:**
  - Lives in a well-maintained household with access to clean water and food.
  - No recent travel or exposure to sick individuals.

## IDEAS, CONCERNS, EXPECTATIONS:

- **Ideas:** Mother suspects that Ahmad's fatigue and poor weight gain are related to him being a fussy eater.
- **Concerns:** Worried that Ahmed's health may deteriorate if there is no improvement.
- **Expectations:** Hopes for a clear diagnosis and a treatment plan.

## ON EXAMINATION:

- **General Appearance:** Thin and pale child with signs of irritability.
- **Growth Parameters:**
  - **Weight:** Below 5th percentile.
  - **Height:** At the 10th percentile.
- **Vital Signs:** Temperature 36.9°C, HR 120 bpm, RR 35 breaths/min, $SpO_2$: 97% on room air.
- **Systemic Examination:**
  - **HEENT:** Pallor, frontal bossing, and maxillary bone prominence noted.
  - **Chest:** Mild tachypnoea, no wheezes or crackles.
  - **Cardiac:** Systolic murmur over the left sternal border.
  - **Abdomen:** Mild hepatosplenomegaly.
  - **Extremities:** No clubbing or cyanosis.

## INVESTIGATIONS:

1. **Radiological Findings:**
   - **X-Ray:** Shows maxillary bone prominence and skull bossing (indicative of extramedullary haematopoiesis).
2. **Diagnostic Tests to Order:**
   - **CBC with differential:** Evaluate haemoglobin levels and red cell indices.
   - **Peripheral blood smear:** Look for microcytic hypochromic anaemia and target cells.
   - **Serum ferritin and iron studies:** Exclude iron deficiency.
   - **Haemoglobin electrophoresis:** Confirm the presence of abnormal haemoglobins (e.g., HbF, HbA2).
   - **Genetic testing:** Identify mutations in the beta-globin gene.

## WHAT IS THE DIAGNOSIS?

**Thalassemia Major (beta-thalassemia).**

Thalassemia major is a serious inherited blood disorder where the body can't produce enough haemoglobin – the protein in red blood cells responsible for carrying oxygen. This deficiency leads to severe anaemia, causing symptoms like fatigue, weakness, pale skin, and slowed growth in children. Individuals with thalassemia major often require regular blood transfusions throughout their lives to manage the condition.

## OUTLINE THE MANAGEMENT PLAN:

*Immediate Steps:*

1. **Refer to a Paediatric Haematologist:**
   - Confirm diagnosis with specialized testing.
   - Plan for regular blood transfusions to maintain haemoglobin levels.
2. **Parental Counselling:**
   - Educate about the nature of thalassemia major, its hereditary basis, and the need for lifelong management.
   - Discuss the importance of routine transfusions and monitoring for complications.
3. **Nutritional Support:**
   - Ensure adequate calorie intake to support growth.
   - Supplement with folic acid (400 mcg/day) to support red blood cell production.

*Long-Term Management:*

1. **Iron Chelation Therapy:**
   - Begin when serum ferritin levels are elevated due to transfusion-related iron overload.
   - Options include deferoxamine or oral chelators.
2. **Monitor for Complications:**
   - Regular cardiac and liver function tests.
   - Growth and developmental assessments.
3. **Genetic Counselling:**
   - Offer genetic screening for parents and siblings.
   - Discuss the risk of recurrence in future pregnancies and prenatal diagnostic options.

## QUESTIONS:

1. **What tests confirm thalassemia major?**
   - CBC, peripheral smear, haemoglobin electrophoresis, and genetic testing for beta-globin mutations.
2. **What are the complications of untreated thalassemia major?**
   - Severe anaemia, growth retardation, organ damage due to iron overload, and skeletal deformities.
3. **What are the goals of iron chelation therapy?**
   - Prevent organ damage (heart, liver) caused by iron overload from repeated transfusions.
4. **How do you distinguish thalassemia major from iron deficiency anaemia?**
   - MCV is very low in thalassemia when compared to HB drop.
   - Serum ferritin/iron studies normal or high in thalassemia; low in iron deficiency.
   - RDW usually normal in thalassemia, raised in iron deficiency.
5. **What genetic counselling should be offered to the parents?**
   - If both are carriers of beta-thalassemia trait, 25% thalassemia trait, 50% being a carrier, 25% of being unaffected.
6. **When iron chelation therapy be started, and what are the options?**
   - When ferritin is persistently >1000 ng/mL or after 10–12 transfusions.
   - Deferoxamine (subcutaneous infusion), Deferasirox (oral), Deferiprone (oral).

CASE 39

# Paediatric Obesity

## Doctor's Notes

*Patient Details:*

- **Name:** Omar Hasan
- **Age:** 13 years
- **Presenting Complaint:** Concern about weight gain
- **Setting:** Family Medicine Clinic

## PATIENT'S SIMULATED SCRIPT:

### Opening Statement:

"I'm worried about my weight. Everyone at school calls me fat."

## HISTORY:

- **Onset of Weight Gain:**
  - Started around 2 years ago, progressively worsening.
- **Associated Symptoms:**
  - Fatigue, feeling cold often.
  - No changes in appetite or eating habits.
  - No polyuria or polydipsia.
- **Family History:**
  - Father has type 2 diabetes and obesity.
  - Mother is overweight.
- **Dietary History:**
  - High consumption of sugary drinks and processed snacks.
  - Prefers fast food over home-cooked meals.

- **Physical Activity:**
  - Rarely engages in outdoor activities or sports.
  - Spends 4–5 hours daily on screens.
- **Psychosocial History:**
  - Bullying at school due to his weight.
  - Poor self-esteem and reluctance to socialize.

## IDEAS, CONCERNS, EXPECTATIONS:

- **Ideas:** Omar feels his weight is out of control and says it's due to big bones.
- **Concerns:** Worries he will continue getting bullied at school.
- **Expectations:** Hopes for medication to help with weight loss.

## ON EXAMINATION:

- **Growth Chart:** Weight is above the 95th percentile for age and height.
- **Vital Signs:** BP 130/85 mmHg, HR 78 bpm, temperature 36.8°C, $SpO_2$ 98% on room air.
- **General Appearance:** Obese adolescent, appearing tired.
- **HEENT:** No goitre.
- **Skin:** Acanthosis nigricans noted on the neck and axillae.
- **Abdomen:** Soft, no organomegaly.
- **Extremities:** No oedema.

## INVESTIGATIONS:

1. **Growth Chart:** BMI >95th percentile for age and sex.
2. **Laboratory Results:**
   - **TSH:** Elevated.
   - **Free T4:** Low (consistent with hypothyroidism).
   - **Fasting Glucose:** 5.8 mmol/L (borderline).
   - **HbA1c:** 5.7% (pre-diabetic range).
   - **Lipid Profile:** Elevated LDL and triglycerides.

## WHAT IS THE DIAGNOSIS?

1. **Obesity** (primary diagnosis).
2. **Hypothyroidism** (likely contributing to weight gain).
3. **Pre-Diabetes.**

## MANAGEMENT PLAN:

*Immediate Steps:*

1. **Address Hypothyroidism:**
   - Start levothyroxine at an appropriate dose based on body weight.
   - Recheck TSH and free T4 in 6–8 weeks.
2. **Lifestyle Modifications for Weight Loss:**
   - **Dietary Advice:**
     - Reduce sugary drinks and processed foods.
     - Increase intake of vegetables, lean proteins, and whole grains.
     - Family-based meal planning to ensure support.

- **Physical Activity:**
  - Encourage at least 60 minutes of moderate activity daily (e.g., walking, swimming).
  - Limit screen time to <2 hours/day.

3. **Psychosocial Support:**
   - Address bullying and self-esteem issues.
   - Refer to a counsellor for behavioural therapy if needed.

*Can He Start Weight-Lowering Drugs?*

- Weight-lowering medications are not first-line treatments in adolescents.
- Consider only if lifestyle interventions fail after 6–12 months and obesity-related complications persist.
- Medications like orlistat are approved for adolescents over 12 but should only be used under specialist supervision.

*Long-Term Management:*

1. **Monitor Weight and BMI:** Regular follow-ups every 2–3 months to assess progress.
2. **Screen for Obesity-Related Complications:**
   - Annual glucose and lipid profile tests.
   - Monitor for hypertension and sleep apnoea.

## QUESTIONS:

1. **What tests should be ordered for an obese child?**
   - TSH and free T4 to assess thyroid function.
   - Fasting glucose and HbA1c to evaluate for diabetes.
   - Lipid profile to check for dyslipidaemia.
   - Liver function tests to rule out non-alcoholic fatty liver disease (NAFLD).
2. **What are the benefits of early weight management in children?**
   - Prevents long-term complications like type 2 diabetes, cardiovascular disease, and joint problems.
   - Improves self-esteem and overall quality of life.
3. **When would you consider pharmacological therapy for paediatric obesity?**
   - Following 6–12 months lifestyle modification with a BMI ≥95th percentile with complications.
4. **Why is acanthosis nigricans clinically relevant?**
   - It implies insulin resistance, which increases the risk of diabetes.

# Post-Streptococcal Glomerulonephritis

CASE 40

## Doctor's Notes

*Patient Details:*

- **Name:** Yousuf Ahmad
- **Age:** 9 years
- **Presenting Complaint:** Swollen eyes
- **Setting:** Family Medicine Clinic

## PATIENT'S SIMULATED SCRIPT:

### Opening Statement:

"My eyes have been puffy for the past few days."

## ARAB BOARD EXPECTATIONS FOR RESIDENT DOCTOR:

- Elicit a detailed history to uncover symptoms suggestive of post-streptococcal glomerulonephritis (PSGN).
- Correlate laboratory results with clinical findings.
- Educate the parents on the condition, its complications, and the management plan.

## HISTORY:

- **Onset of Symptoms:**
  - Swelling started 3 days ago, particularly noticeable around the eyes in the morning.
- **Associated Symptoms:**
  - History of sore throat approximately 2 weeks ago, now resolved.
  - Dark-coloured urine ("tea-coloured") for the past few days.
  - Reduced urine output.
  - Fatigue and lethargy.
  - No fever, skin rashes, joint pain, or abdominal pain.

- **Past Medical History:**
  - No similar episodes in the past.
  - No known allergies or chronic medical conditions.
- **Drug History:**
  - Took paracetamol for sore throat symptoms previously.
  - No regular medications.
- **Family History:**
  - No family history of kidney disease or autoimmune conditions.
- **Lifestyle and Social History:**
  - Active, attends school regularly.
  - No recent travel or exposure to unusual environmental factors.

## IDEAS, CONCERNS, EXPECTATIONS:

- **Ideas:** Parents suspect the swelling may be linked to an eye infection.
- **Concerns:** They are worried it could affect his eyesight.
- **Expectations:** Parents hope for a clear explanation and reassurance that it can be treated.

## ON EXAMINATION:

- **General Appearance:** Child appears well but tired, with noticeable periorbital swelling.
- **Vital Signs:** BP 130/85 mmHg (elevated for age), HR 88 bpm, temperature 36.9°C, $SpO_2$: 98% on room air.
- **Oedema:** Mild, mostly around the eyes; no peripheral oedema.
- **Chest Examination:** Clear breath sounds, no crepitations.
- **Abdomen:** Soft, non-tender; no organomegaly.

## INVESTIGATIONS:

1. **Blood Tests:**
   - **High Anti-Streptolysin O (ASO) titre:** Elevated.
   - **Serum Creatinine:** Slightly elevated.
   - **Blood Urea Nitrogen (BUN):** Elevated.
   - **Serum Complement C3:** Low.
   - Normal liver function tests and electrolytes.
2. **Urinalysis:**
   - Haematuria (microscopic and macroscopic).
   - Proteinuria (mild).
   - No casts or white blood cells.
3. **Other Tests:**
   - **Throat Swab Culture:** Previously positive for Group A Streptococcus.

## WHAT IS THE DIAGNOSIS?

**Post-Streptococcal Glomerulonephritis (PSGN).**

PSGN is a kidney condition that can develop after an infection with certain strains of Streptococcus bacteria, such as strep throat or skin infections.

## OUTLINE THE MANAGEMENT PLAN:

*Immediate Steps:*

1. **Monitor and Manage Blood Pressure:**
   - Prescribe antihypertensives if required (e.g., amlodipine for symptomatic hypertension).
2. **Manage Fluid Retention:**
   - Sodium and fluid restriction.
   - Diuretics (e.g., furosemide) if there are signs of fluid overload.
3. **Symptomatic Relief:**
   - Rest and ensure adequate hydration within restrictions.

*Long-Term Management:*

1. **Monitor Renal Function:**
   - Repeat renal function tests and urinalysis in 1–2 weeks.
2. **Educate Parents:**
   - Explain the condition and reassure that most children recover fully.
   - Emphasize the importance of follow-up to monitor for complications.
3. **Prevent Recurrence:**
   - Encourage timely treatment of future throat infections with antibiotics.

## SAFETY NETTING:

- Advise parents to return or seek urgent care if:
  - Swelling worsens or spreads.
  - Child becomes increasingly fatigued, develops severe headache, or has changes in urine output.

## QUESTIONS:

1. **What tests should be ordered for suspected post-streptococcal glomerulonephritis?**
   - Anti-streptolysin O (ASO) titre.
   - Serum complement levels (e.g., C3).
   - Renal function tests (e.g., creatinine, BUN).
   - Urinalysis.
2. **What are potential complications of PSGN?**
   - Acute kidney injury.
   - Hypertension.
   - Rarely, progression to chronic kidney disease.
3. **What are some "population level" prevention initiatives?**
   - Treat streptococcal pharyngitis promptly, improve hygiene, and educate about early recognition.
4. **How effective is early treatment in preventing PSGN?**
   - Early antibiotic treatment reduces risk by 50–60%.

# CASE 41
# Henoch-Schönlein Purpura

## Doctor's Notes

*Patient Details:*

- **Name:** Omar Hassan
- **Age:** 6 years
- **Presenting Complaint:** Abdominal pain and skin rash
- **Setting:** Family Medicine Clinic

## PATIENT'S SIMULATED SCRIPT:

### Opening Statement:

"My tummy hurts, and this rash showed up yesterday."

## HISTORY:

- **Onset of Symptoms:**
  - Abdominal pain started 2 days ago, intermittent, and located around the umbilical area.
  - Rash appeared yesterday on the lower limbs.
- **Associated Symptoms:**
  - Joint pain in the knees and ankles started 4 days ago, mild and resolved spontaneously.
  - Viral upper respiratory tract infection (URTI) 8 days ago with a runny nose and low-grade fever, now resolved.
  - No vomiting, diarrhoea, or urinary symptoms.
- **Past Medical History:**
  - No previous similar episodes.
  - No known chronic conditions or allergies.
- **Family History:**
  - No family history of autoimmune diseases or bleeding disorders.
- **Lifestyle and Social History:**
  - Active child, attends school regularly.
  - No recent travel or contact with sick individuals.

## IDEAS, CONCERNS, EXPECTATIONS:

- **Ideas:** Parents think he's probably got a new chest infection.
- **Concerns:** Worried the rash may be a sign of something serious like meningitis.
- **Expectations:** Hope for reassurance and effective treatment.

## ON EXAMINATION:

- **General Appearance:** Child appears well but slightly irritable.
- **Vital Signs:** BP 95/60 mmHg, HR: 96 bpm, temperature 37.2°C, $SpO_2$ 98% on room air.
- **Abdominal Examination:**
  - Mild tenderness around the umbilical area.
  - No guarding or rebound tenderness.
  - Bowel sounds present.
- **Skin Examination:**
  - Non-blanching purpuric rash on the lower limbs and buttocks.
- **Joint Examination:**
  - No active swelling, erythema, or tenderness.
  - Full range of motion in all joints.

## INVESTIGATIONS:

- Blood Tests:
  - **CBC:** Normal platelet count, no evidence of thrombocytopenia.
  - **CRP/ESR:** Mildly elevated, consistent with inflammation.
  - **Renal Function Tests:** Normal.
- Urinalysis:
  - Presence of microscopic haematuria.
  - No proteinuria.

Please utilise online database to visualise an image for a simulated objective structured clinical examination (OSCE). Numerous sites, including dermnet.nz.

## WHAT IS THE DIAGNOSIS?

**Henoch-Schönlein Purpura (HSP).**

HSP is a condition that causes inflammation in small blood vessels, leading to symptoms like a purplish rash (usually on the legs and buttocks), joint pain, stomach pain, and sometimes kidney issues. It is often triggered by an infection, such as a cold or sore throat, and usually affects children.

In simple terms, it is as if the body's immune system gets confused after fighting an infection and causes swelling in the tiny blood vessels. Most children recover completely, but some might need closer monitoring if their kidneys are affected.

## HOW WOULD YOU MANAGE THIS PATIENT?

*Immediate Steps:*

1. **Symptomatic Management:**
   - Provide paracetamol for pain relief as needed.
   - Encourage hydration and a bland diet to minimize abdominal discomfort.

2. **Monitor for Complications:**
    - Educate caregivers to watch for worsening abdominal pain (intussusception risk), vomiting, or blood in stool.
    - Monitor urine output and appearance for signs of nephritis.
3. **Reassurance and Education:**
    - Explain that HSP is self-limiting in most cases and resolves in a few weeks.
    - Emphasize the importance of follow-up for urine checks to rule out kidney involvement.

*Long-Term Management:*

1. **Follow-up:**
    - Weekly urinalysis for 1 month, then biweekly for 3 months, and monthly for 6 months.
2. **Referral:**
    - Refer to a paediatric for further evaluation. Clinically we would refer if there were signs of significant renal involvement (e.g., persistent haematuria, proteinuria, or hypertension).

## SAFETY NETTING:

- Advise parents to seek urgent care if:
    - Abdominal pain becomes severe or localized.
    - Rash spreads or worsens significantly.
    - Symptoms such as swelling, joint pain, or haematuria persist or worsen.

## QUESTIONS:

1. **What are the common complications of HSP?**
    - Gastrointestinal complications such as intussusception.
    - Renal involvement, including haematuria, proteinuria, and nephritis.
    - Rarely, chronic kidney disease in severe cases.
2. **How do you monitor renal involvement in HSP?**
    - Regular urinalysis to check for haematuria and proteinuria.
    - Blood pressure monitoring to detect hypertension.

Follow-up in a new case of HSP is crucial to monitor for potential complications, especially kidney involvement.

## A GENERAL GUIDELINE:

**Initial Follow-up Schedule:**

1. **First Week After Diagnosis:**
    - Reassess symptoms (rash, abdominal pain, joint pain).
    - Check blood pressure and urine for signs of kidney involvement (protein or blood).
2. **Weekly for the First Month:**
    - Monitor for any new symptoms or worsening of existing ones.
    - Continue blood pressure checks and urine tests.
3. **Every 2–4 Weeks for the Next 6 Months:**
    - Focus on kidney health, as complications like nephritis can develop later.
    - Check urine for proteinuria or haematuria and monitor blood pressure.
4. **As Needed:**
    - If kidney involvement is detected, follow up more frequently with a nephrologist.
    - If symptoms resolve completely and no kidney issues arise, the frequency of follow-up can be reduced.

**Red Flags to Seek Immediate Care:**

- Severe abdominal pain, vomiting, or blood in the stool.
- Signs of worsening kidney function (swelling, reduced urine output).
- High blood pressure readings.

**What is the pathophysiology of HSP?**

IgA immune complex deposition in small vessels leads to leukocytoclastic vasculitis affecting skin, GI tract, joints, and kidneys.

**What are the gastrointestinal complications of HSP?**

Intussusception, GI bleeding, bowel ischaemia, and perforation.

**What is the typical prognosis of HSP in children?**

Self resolution within 6 weeks, with long-term kidney damage being quite rare.

# CASE 42

# Developmental Delay – Speech

## Doctor's Notes

*Patient Details:*

- **Name:** Abdullah
- **Age:** 4 years
- **Presenting Complaint:** Concern about delayed speech
- **Setting:** Family Medicine Clinic

## PATIENT'S SIMULATED SCRIPT:

### Opening Statement:

"I'm worried about my child's speech development."

## HISTORY:

- **Speech Development:**
  - Speaks in one- to two-word phrases; lags behind peers in vocabulary and sentence formation.
  - Difficulty pronouncing words clearly.
- **Hearing History:**
  - Repeated episodes of acute otitis media since infancy.
  - Parental observation of child not responding to soft sounds or when called from another room.
- **Other Developmental Milestones:**
  - Walking, running, and fine motor skills are age appropriate.
  - Socially interacts with family members but sometimes appears inattentive.
- **Birth and Neonatal History:**
  - Full-term delivery, no complications.
  - No history of neonatal jaundice or other illnesses.
- **Family and Social History:**
  - No family history of hearing loss or speech delays.
  - Lives with both parents, no significant stressors in the household.

- **Lifestyle History:**
  - Attends preschool but struggles to communicate with peers.
  - Watches TV and listens to music but prefers visual over verbal instructions.

## IDEAS, CONCERNS, EXPECTATIONS:

- **Ideas:** The parents attribute this to a possible hereditary factor, as the child's father had delayed speech development during childhood.
- **Concerns:** Worried that he may have autism or something similar.
- **Expectations:** Hope for reassurance and effective treatment.

## PAST MEDICAL HISTORY:

- Recurrent acute otitis media (approximately five to six episodes per year).
- No known allergies.

## DRUG HISTORY:

- None currently.
- Previous antibiotic treatments for otitis media.

## INVESTIGATIONS AND SCREENING:

- **Audiogram and Tympanometry:**
  - Bilateral conductive hearing loss.
- **M-CHAT Screening Score:**
  - Score: 1 (low risk for autism spectrum disorder).

## ON EXAMINATION:

- **General Appearance:** Alert and interactive.
- **Growth Parameters:** Normal for age.
- **ENT Examination:**
  - Tympanic membranes appear dull bilaterally, with evidence of effusion.
  - No acute redness or perforation.

## WHAT IS THE DIAGNOSIS?

- **Speech Delay** secondary to conductive hearing loss.
- **Likely Chronic Otitis Media with Effusion** (glue ear).

## OUTLINE THE MANAGEMENT FOR THIS PATIENT:

1. ***Referral to ENT Specialist:***
   - Evaluate for potential surgical intervention, such as tympanostomy tube placement (grommets), to address middle ear effusion.
2. ***Speech and Language Therapy:***
   - Early initiation to improve language skills and catch up developmentally.

3. ***Hearing Support:***
   - Temporary hearing aids, if deemed necessary by the ENT specialist, until surgical intervention.
4. ***Parental Guidance and Support:***
   - Encourage speaking to the child in short, clear sentences and engaging in interactive activities (e.g., reading books together).
   - Minimize background noise at home to help with hearing.
5. ***Regular Follow-up:***
   - Monitor speech and hearing development after intervention.
   - Repeat audiometry and tympanometry in 3–6 months to assess progress.

## QUESTIONS:

1. **What are the complications of untreated conductive hearing loss in children?**
   - Persistent speech and language delays.
   - Learning difficulties due to impaired communication.
   - Social isolation and behavioural issues.
2. **What does a low-risk M-CHAT score mean?**
   - It indicates that the child is unlikely to have autism spectrum disorder, though further monitoring is essential if other concerns arise.
3. **What is the role of tympanostomy tubes (grommets) in this setting?**
   - Drainage of middle ear effusions helps in restoring normal hearing, which helps support normal speech and language development.

# CASE 43 Chickenpox

## Doctor's Notes

*Patient Details:*

- **Name:** Ahmad
- **Age:** 4 years
- **Presenting Complaint:** Fever and skin rash
- **Setting:** Family Medicine Clinic

## PATIENT'S SIMULATED SCRIPT:

### Opening Statement:

"He's been having a fever and this rash appeared a couple of days ago."

## HISTORY:

- **History of Presenting Complaint:**
  - Rash started as red spots and turned into blisters.
  - Fever (38.5°C) began 2 days before the rash appeared.
  - Mild itchiness noted but no severe discomfort.
  - No difficulty in breathing or severe lethargy.
- **Past Medical History:**
  - Otherwise healthy.
  - Vaccination status up to date except for chickenpox vaccine (not given).
- **Family and Social History:**
  - Pregnant mother in her 15th week of gestation.
  - Child attends day-care regularly.
- **Drug History:**
  - No regular medications.
  - No known drug allergies.

## IDEAS, CONCERNS, EXPECTATIONS:

- **Ideas:** The parent suspects it could be a skin infection.
- **Concerns:** The mother is worried about the child's diagnosis and potential need for admission, and is concerned that the illness may have affected her pregnancy.
- **Expectations:** Seeks advice on managing the child's symptoms and ensuring the mother and unborn baby are safe.

## ON EXAMINATION:

- **Vital Signs:**
  - Temp: 38.5°C
  - HR: 92 bpm
  - RR: 20 breaths/min
  - BP: Normal for age
- **General Appearance:** Alert and interactive.
- **Skin:** Vesicular rash in various stages of healing, primarily on the trunk and face.
- **ENT:** Normal.
- **Chest and Cardiovascular:** Normal.
- **Abdomen:** Soft and non-tender.
- **Neurological Exam:** Normal.

## INVESTIGATIONS:

1. **Child's Serology:**
   - Not required, as the clinical picture is consistent with chickenpox.
2. **Mother's Serology:**
   - VZV IgM: Negative.
   - VZV IgG: 130 (below protective threshold of 150).

## DIAGNOSIS:

1. **Child:** Chickenpox (varicella).
2. **Mother:** Non-immune to varicella (at risk).

Chickenpox is a highly contagious illness caused by the varicella-zoster virus. It leads to an itchy rash with small, fluid-filled blisters, often starting on the chest, back, and face, then spreading to other parts of the body.

## OUTLINE THE MANAGEMENT PLAN FOR BOTH THE CHILD AND THE PREGNANT WOMAN:

*For the Child:*

1. **Symptomatic Management:**
   - Paracetamol for fever (AVOID NSAIDs!!!).
   - Calamine lotion or antihistamines for itching.
   - Maintain hydration.
   - Avoid scratching to prevent secondary bacterial infection.
   - Advise isolation until all lesions crust over (approximately 5–7 days).
2. **Follow-up:**
   - Advise to return if the child develops any complications (e.g., high fever, difficulty breathing, or signs of secondary bacterial infection).

*For the Pregnant Mother:*

1. **Immediate Management:**
    - Administer varicella-zoster immune globulin (VZIG) as soon as possible (within 10 days of exposure) due to IgG levels below the protective threshold of 150.
    - Provide reassurance about the efficacy of VZIG in reducing the risk of maternal varicella.
2. **Monitoring:**
    - Observe for signs of varicella infection in the mother (rash, fever) despite VZIG administration.
    - Repeat VZV IgG testing in 2–4 weeks if needed.
3. **Education:**
    - Advise avoiding close contact with the child until all lesions have crusted over.
    - Counsel about symptoms of varicella and when to seek medical attention.

*Preventive Measures:*

- Recommend vaccination for close family contacts (if not pregnant or immunocompromised) to prevent future episodes.

## QUESTIONS:

1. **What are the complications of chickenpox?**
    - Secondary bacterial infection of the skin, pneumonia, encephalitis, and dehydration.
2. **What are the benefits of VZIG for the mother?**
    - It reduces the risk of developing severe varicella infection and potential complications for both mother and foetus.
3. **When should antiviral therapy be considered in varicella?**
    - With severe and complicated cases, immunocompromised children, pregnancy, and patients with pneumonia or encephalitis.

CASE 44

# Gastroesophageal Reflux Disease

## Doctor's Notes

*Patient Details:*

- **Name:** Ahmed Yasin
- **Age:** 14 years
- **Occupation:** Student
- **Presenting Complaint:** Complaining of heartburn and acid reflux
- **Setting:** Family Medicine Clinic

## PATIENT'S SIMULATED SCRIPT:

### Opening Statement:

"I keep getting this burning feeling in my chest after eating."

## HISTORY:

- **Present Illness:**
  - Complains of heartburn and sour taste in the mouth, especially after meals.
  - Symptoms started 2 months ago, occurring three to four times a week.
  - Aggravated by lying down after consuming spicy/fatty foods.
  - Relieved partially by drinking water or standing up.
- **Associated Symptoms:**
  - Occasional nausea but no vomiting.
  - No weight loss, fever, or night sweats.
  - No difficulty swallowing or blood in vomit/stools.
- **Past Medical History:**
  - No known chronic illnesses.
  - Recurrent tonsillitis during childhood, treated with antibiotics.

- **Drug History:**
  - Takes over-the-counter antacids occasionally with some relief.
  - No known allergies.
- **Family History:**
  - Father has peptic ulcer disease.
  - Mother has type 2 diabetes.
- **Lifestyle and Social History:**
  - Consumes junk food and carbonated drinks frequently.
  - Skips meals, especially breakfast.
  - Sedentary lifestyle with limited physical activity.
  - No smoking or alcohol use.

## IDEAS, CONCERNS, EXPECTATIONS:

- **Ideas:** Thinks he may have an infection in his stomach. His neighbour had something similar and was prescribed antibiotics.
- **Concerns:** Worries the condition might be serious or long-lasting.
- **Expectations:** Hopes for quick relief and guidance on how to prevent the symptoms.

## ON EXAMINATION:

- **General Appearance:** Alert and well-appearing.
- **Vital Signs:**
  - BP: 110/70 mmHg
  - HR: 78 bpm
  - Temp: 36.8°C
  - $SpO_2$: 98% on room air
- **Abdomen:**
  - Soft and non-tender.
  - No organomegaly or palpable masses.
- **Respiratory and Cardiovascular Examination:** Normal findings.

## INVESTIGATIONS AND RESULTS:

1. **Lifestyle Assessment:** Diet rich in processed foods; irregular meal patterns.
2. **Blood Work (if requested):**
   - **CBC:** Normal.
   - **CRP:** Normal.
3. **Further Tests (if considered):**
   - No immediate endoscopy required unless red flags (e.g., weight loss, dysphagia) develop.

## WHAT IS THE DIAGNOSIS?

**Gastroesophageal Reflux Disease (GERD).**

GERD is a chronic condition where stomach acid frequently flows back into the oesophagus – the tube connecting the mouth and stomach. This backwash, or acid reflux, irritates the oesophageal lining, leading to symptoms like heartburn – a burning sensation in the chest – and regurgitation of food or sour liquid.

## OUTLINE THE MANAGEMENT PLAN:

*Immediate Steps:*

1. **Lifestyle Modifications:**
   - Avoid trigger foods (spicy, fatty, or acidic foods; carbonated drinks; caffeine).
   - Eat smaller, more frequent meals and avoid eating 2–3 hours before bedtime.
   - Elevate the head of the bed while sleeping.
   - Encourage weight reduction if overweight.
2. **Pharmacological Management:**
   - Start a proton pump inhibitor (e.g., omeprazole 20 mg once daily for 4–8 weeks).
   - Continue using antacids as needed for breakthrough symptoms.
3. **Counselling and Education:**
   - Educate on the importance of healthy eating habits and regular physical activity.
   - Discuss the need to reduce junk food and include more fruits, vegetables, and whole grains.

*Follow-up:*

- Review in 4 weeks to assess symptom improvement.
- If symptoms persist or worsen, consider referral for further investigation (e.g., upper GI endoscopy).

## SAFETY NETTING:

Advise to return or seek urgent care if:
- Symptoms worsen or new symptoms such as difficulty swallowing or weight loss develop.
- Vomiting blood or passing black stools occurs.

## QUESTIONS:

1. **What are the common causes of GERD in adolescents?**
   - Poor diet, obesity, stress, or anatomical factors such as hiatal hernia.
2. **What are the complications of untreated GERD?**
   - Oesophagitis, strictures, Barrett oesophagus, or increased risk of oesophageal cancer.
3. **How does a proton pump inhibitor (PPI) work in GERD?**
   - PPIs inhibit the H+/K+ ATPase pump in gastric parietal cells, reducing acid secretion and allowing mucosal healing.

CASE 45

# Recurrent Urinary Tract Infection

## Doctor's Notes

*Patient Details:*

- **Name:** Huda Ali
- **Age:** 5 years
- **Presenting Complaint:** Recurrent urinary tract infections (UTIs)
- **Setting:** Family Medicine Clinic

## PATIENT'S SIMULATED SCRIPT:

### Opening Statement by parent:

"Her urine infections keep coming back, and I don't know why."

## HISTORY:

- **Present Illness:**
  - Complains of recurrent UTIs over the past 5 weeks.
  - Symptoms include fever, abdominal pain, and foul-smelling urine during episodes.
  - Last episode was 1 week ago. Treated with antibiotics, but she did not complete the prescribed course.
  - Currently asymptomatic but concerned about recurrence.
- **Associated Symptoms:**
  - Occasionally complains of lower abdominal pain.
  - No vomiting or diarrhoea.
  - No weight loss or loss of appetite.
- **Past Medical History:**
  - Two episodes of confirmed UTI within the last 5 weeks.
  - Antibiotics were prescribed but not completed during both episodes because the patient found the antibiotic that was prescribed (erythromycin) to be "yucky" so did not complete either course.
  - No history of structural kidney issues identified previously.

- **Drug History:**
  - Used prescribed antibiotics for UTIs but did not complete the courses.
  - No known drug allergies.
- **Family History:**
  - Mother had recurrent UTIs in childhood but no long-term complications.
  - No family history of kidney disease or structural abnormalities.
- **Social History:**
  - Lives with parents and two siblings.
  - Attends school, developmentally appropriate for age.
  - Drinks mostly sugary drinks, limited water intake.

## IDEAS, CONCERNS, EXPECTATIONS:

- **Ideas:** Mother thinks the child might be holding her urine, because Mother read on a Facebook post that that causes urine infections.
- **Concerns:** Mother is worried she will have to make repeated doctor visits until the child stops getting UTIs.
- **Expectations:** Hopes for a solution to prevent further infections.

## ON EXAMINATION:

- **General Appearance:** Active, alert child.
- **Vital Signs:**
  - BP: 92/58 mmHg
  - HR: 100 bpm
  - Temp: 36.7°C
  - $SpO_2$: 99% on room air
- **Abdomen:**
  - Soft, non-tender.
  - No palpable masses or organomegaly.
- **Genital Examination:** Normal external genitalia, no signs of redness or discharge.
- **Growth:** Normal for age; height and weight within the 25th percentile.

## INVESTIGATIONS AND RESULTS:

1. **Urinalysis:**
   - No current infection; clear urine.
   - No haematuria or proteinuria.
2. **Urine Culture** (from previous infections):
   - *E. coli* sensitive to nitrofurantoin and cefixime.
3. **Ultrasound:**
   - Hydronephrosis with a ureterocoele.
   - Poor echogenicity of one kidney, suggestive of potential scarring or dysfunction.

## WHAT IS THE DIAGNOSIS?

1. **Recurrent Urinary Tract Infections** with incomplete antibiotic treatment.
2. **Hydronephrosis and Ureterocoele** with evidence of kidney damage.

Recurrent UTIs (experiencing multiple episodes of UTIs over a certain period) – specifically defined as having two or more infections within 6 months or three or more within a year. UTIs occur when bacteria enter the urinary tract, leading to symptoms like a strong urge to urinate, a burning sensation during urination, and cloudy or strong-smelling urine.

## OUTLINE THE MANAGEMENT PLAN:

*Immediate Steps:*

1. **Treatment of Current UTI (if infection confirmed):**
   - Prescribe antibiotics based on culture sensitivity:
     - **Nitrofurantoin**: 5–7 mg/kg/day divided into 2 doses for 7–10 days.
   - Ensure parents are educated on the importance of completing the antibiotic course.
2. **Preventive Measures:**
   - Start prophylactic antibiotics to prevent recurrence:
     - **Trimethoprim:** 2 mg/kg once daily or
     - **Nitrofurantoin:** 1 mg/kg once daily.
   - Educate on proper hydration and frequent voiding to reduce UTI risk.
3. **Referral and Further Investigations:**
   - Refer to a paediatric nephrologist or urologist for further evaluation and management of hydronephrosis and ureterocele.
   - Consider performing a voiding cystourethrogram (VCUG) to evaluate for vesicoureteral reflux (VUR).
   - Perform a renal scan (DMSA) to assess the extent of kidney scarring and function.

*Long-Term Management:*

1. Monitor renal function with regular blood tests (e.g., creatinine, GFR).
2. Periodic urinalysis and urine cultures to detect asymptomatic bacteriuria or recurrent infections.
3. Continue follow-ups with nephrology or urology for potential surgical intervention (e.g., ureterocoele excision).

## SAFETY NETTING:

- Advise parents to bring the child back if:
  - She develops fever, abdominal pain, or signs of a UTI.
  - There is difficulty tolerating the antibiotics.

## QUESTIONS:

1. **How do you manage recurrent UTIs in children?**
   - Treat acute infections with antibiotics based on culture sensitivity.
   - Prevent recurrence with prophylactic antibiotics, adequate hydration, and addressing underlying causes (e.g., structural abnormalities).
2. **What is the recommended duration of antibiotics for UTI in children?**
   - Typically 7–10 days for acute infections, depending on severity and age.
3. **What complications can hydronephrosis and ureterocoele cause?**
   - Renal scarring, reduced kidney function, and chronic kidney disease.
4. **What are the definitions of recurrent UTI and complicated UTI in children, and how do they influence management?**
   - **Recurrent UTI:** Greater than or equal to two febrile UTIs in 6 months, or three in a year.
   - **Complicated UTI:** UTI associated with structural/functional abnormality, obstruction, or renal scarring.

# CASE 46
# Panic Attack

## Doctor's Notes

*Patient Details:*

- **Name:** Ahmed Salman
- **Age:** 30 years
- **Occupation:** Marketing executive
- **Presenting Complaint:** Concerns about recurrent episodes of fast heart rate and associated symptoms
- **Setting:** Family Medicine Clinic

## PATIENT'S SIMULATED SCRIPT:

### Opening Statement:

"I'm here to discuss the results of the tests I had after those heart episodes."

## HISTORY:

- **History of Present Illness:**
  - Reports experiencing sudden episodes of rapid heart rate, lasting 10–20 minutes.
  - Associated symptoms include shortness of breath, sweating, dizziness, and a sense of impending doom.
  - Episodes occur unexpectedly, even during rest.
  - No identifiable triggers, although episodes are more frequent during stressful periods at work.
  - No chest pain, fainting, or lasting weakness after episodes.
- **Past Medical History:**
  - No known chronic illnesses.
  - No history of cardiovascular or thyroid disease.
- **Drug History:**
  - Occasionally uses paracetamol for headaches.
  - No regular medications or known drug allergies.

- **Family History:**
  - Father has hypertension and type 2 diabetes.
  - No family history of cardiac arrhythmias or psychiatric disorders.
- **Social History:**
  - Non-smoker and non-alcoholic.
  - Exercises occasionally, but recent episodes have made him avoid physical activity.
- **Lifestyle:**
  - High-stress job with frequent deadlines.
  - Sleeps 5–6 hours per night but reports difficulty falling asleep due to worrying.

## IDEAS, CONCERNS, EXPECTATIONS:

- **Ideas:** Believes he might have a heart problem, possibly arrhythmia.
- **Concerns:** Fears that these episodes could lead to a heart attack or other serious complications.
- **Expectations:** Wants reassurance and a treatment plan to prevent future episodes.

## ON EXAMINATION:

- **General Appearance:** Alert, anxious demeanour.
- **Vital Signs:**
  - BP: 120/80 mmHg
  - HR: 76 bpm, regular
  - Temp: 36.7°C
  - $SpO_2$: 98% on room air
- **Systemic Examination:**
  - **Cardiovascular:** Normal heart sounds, no murmurs or irregularities.
  - **Respiratory:** Clear chest bilaterally.
  - **Neurological:** No focal neurological deficits.
  - **Thyroid:** No palpable goitre or nodules.

## INVESTIGATIONS AND RESULTS:

- **ECG (performed during the last visit):** Normal sinus rhythm with no abnormalities.
- **Thyroid Function Tests:** TSH and free T4 within normal limits.
- **Complete Blood Count:** Normal.

## WHAT IS THE DIAGNOSIS?

**Panic Disorder.**

Panic disorder is a mental health condition characterized by sudden and repeated episodes of intense fear, known as panic attacks, that occur unexpectedly and without an obvious trigger.

## OUTLINE THE MANAGEMENT PLAN:

*Explanation and Reassurance:*

1. **Diagnosis Discussion:**
   - Explain that his episodes are consistent with panic disorder and not due to a cardiac issue.
   - Reassure him that his heart is healthy based on the ECG and other tests.

*Immediate Steps:*

2. **Lifestyle Modifications:**
   - Practice stress management techniques such as deep breathing exercises, yoga, or meditation.
   - Regular physical activity tailored to his comfort level.
   - Ensure 7–8 hours of sleep by establishing a consistent bedtime routine.
3. **Psychological Support:**
   - Recommend referral to a psychologist for cognitive-behavioural therapy (CBT), which is proven effective in managing panic disorder.
4. **Medication (if required):**
   - Consider short-term use of a selective serotonin reuptake inhibitor (SSRI) such as sertraline if episodes are frequent or disabling.
   - Discuss risks, benefits, and side effects before initiation.

*Long-Term Management:*

5. **Follow-up Plan:**
   - Schedule a review in 2–4 weeks to assess symptoms and response to therapy.
   - Monitor for side effects of medication if started.

## QUESTIONS:

1. **What are the common symptoms of panic disorder?**
   - Sudden onset of intense fear, rapid heart rate, sweating, shortness of breath, dizziness, and a sense of impending doom.
2. **What are the treatment options for panic disorder?**
   - **Non-pharmacological:** Lifestyle changes, stress management, and CBT.
   - **Pharmacological:** SSRIs or benzodiazepines for short-term use in severe cases.
   - Be knowledgeable of some dosages and how to initiate; for example, Sertraline 50 mg once daily for 4 weeks then reassess if not improving symptoms (earlier if worsening symptoms).
3. **What are the first-line pharmacological options, dosing, and escalation strategy for panic disorder?**
   - **SSRIs:** Sertraline (start 25–50 mg daily, titrate to 100–200 mg if needed).
   - **SNRIs:** Venlafaxine XR (start 37.5 mg, titrate up to 225 mg).
   - **Benzodiazepines:** e.g., clonazepam (0.25–0.5 mg BID) *only short-term bridge* while waiting for SSRI effect.
   - **Escalation:** Reassess after 4–6 weeks; if partial response, uptitrate SSRI dose. If no response, switch class (SSRI → SNRI) or augment with CBT.
4. **How would you counsel a patient reluctant to accept a psychiatric diagnosis?**
   - **Normalize symptoms:** "These are real physical symptoms, but they're due to the body's fight-or-flight response."
   - **Emphasize diagnosis of exclusion:** cardiac, thyroid, and blood tests are normal.
   - Explain that CBT and SSRIs are actually treatments that aid the brain's stress wiring, rather than referring to the condition as a mental illness.

CASE

# Anxiety and Insomnia 47

## Doctor's Notes

*Patient Details:*

- **Name:** Khalid Ahmed
- **Age:** 24 years
- **Occupation:** University student
- **Presenting Complaint:** Follow-up for generalized anxiety and worsening symptoms
- **Setting:** Family Medicine Clinic

## PATIENT'S SIMULATED SCRIPT:

### Opening Statement:

"I feel like my anxiety is getting worse, and I can't sleep properly."

## HISTORY:

- **History of Present Illness:**
  - Initial visit: Scored 6 on GAD-7, mild generalized anxiety with symptoms of restlessness, occasional difficulty concentrating, and mild irritability.
  - Current visit: Scored 18 on GAD-7, indicating severe anxiety. Reports persistent worry about daily activities and feeling on edge most of the time.
  - Symptoms worsen at night, with racing thoughts preventing him from falling asleep.
  - Describes physical symptoms such as palpitations, chest tightness, muscle tension, and frequent headaches.
- **Sleep Disturbances:**
  - Difficulty falling asleep and staying asleep, resulting in 4–5 hours of sleep per night.
  - Feels fatigued and less productive during the day.
- **Triggers:**
  - Reports academic pressure, social expectations, and fear of failure.
  - No recent traumatic events, substance use, or significant lifestyle changes.

- **Past Medical History:**
  - None significant.
  - No history of depression, panic attacks, or other psychiatric illnesses.
- **Drug History:**
  - Occasionally takes paracetamol for headaches.
  - No regular medications or known allergies.
- **Family History:**
  - Mother has generalized anxiety disorder and hypothyroidism.
  - Father has hypertension.
- **Social History:**
  - Non-smoker, occasional coffee drinker (three to four cups/week).
  - Lives with family and has supportive parents but feels overwhelmed by their expectations.
- **Lifestyle:**
  - Does not exercise regularly.
  - Eats irregular meals, often skipping breakfast.

## IDEAS, CONCERNS, EXPECTATIONS:

- **Ideas:** Believes he may have a more serious mental health condition or a physical illness causing these symptoms.
- **Concerns:** Fears that his anxiety may lead to long-term health problems or failure in academics.
- **Expectations:** Hopes for a treatment plan to manage anxiety and improve his sleep.

## ON EXAMINATION:

- **General Appearance:** Appears anxious and fatigued.
- **Vital Signs:**
  - BP: 122/76 mmHg
  - HR: 88 bpm, regular
  - Temp: 36.8°C
  - $SpO_2$: 98% on room air
- **Systemic Examination:**
  - **Cardiovascular:** Normal heart sounds, no murmurs.
  - **Respiratory:** Clear chest bilaterally.
  - **Neurological:** No focal deficits.
  - **Thyroid:** No palpable goitre or tenderness.

## INVESTIGATIONS:

1. **GAD-7 Score:** 18 (severe anxiety).
2. **Thyroid Function Tests:** Pending but indicated due to family history.
3. **CBC, Vitamin B12, and Folate Levels:** Pending to rule out anaemia or deficiencies contributing to fatigue and insomnia.

## WHAT IS THE DIAGNOSIS?

1. **Generalized Anxiety Disorder (Primary Diagnosis)** – Based on persistent and excessive worry with a high GAD-7 score.
2. **Insomnia Disorder** – Likely secondary to anxiety, but primary insomnia should be ruled out.
3. **Hyperthyroidism or Hypothyroidism** – To be ruled out with TSH and T4 testing given family history and overlapping symptoms.

4. **Major Depressive Disorder** – Consider if low mood or loss of interest persists beyond 2 weeks.
5. **Panic Disorder** – Rule out based on episodic nature and additional symptoms of panic attacks.

Generalized anxiety disorder (GAD) is a mental health condition characterized by persistent and excessive worry about various aspects of daily life, such as health, work, or family, even when there is little or no reason to worry. This ongoing anxiety can interfere with daily activities and relationships.

## MANAGEMENT PLAN:

*Immediate Steps:*

1. **Lifestyle Modifications:**
   - Reduce caffeine intake to no more than 1 cup/day, especially in the afternoon and evening.
   - Encourage physical activity (e.g., 30 minutes of walking daily) to help reduce anxiety and improve sleep.
   - Establish a consistent sleep routine, avoiding screen time 1 hour before bed.
2. **Psychological Therapy:**
   - Refer for cognitive-behavioural therapy (CBT) to address anxiety triggers and teach relaxation techniques.
3. **Medication (if required):**
   - Consider starting a selective serotonin reuptake inhibitor (SSRI) such as sertraline, starting with a low dose (e.g., 25–50 mg daily).
   - For insomnia:
     - Short-term use of melatonin 2–5 mg at bedtime.
     - Avoid benzodiazepines unless symptoms are debilitating.

*Long-Term Management:*

4. **Monitoring:**
   - Schedule follow-up in 2–4 weeks to assess response to therapy and medication if started.
   - Monitor for side effects of medication, especially during the first few weeks.
5. **Investigations:**
   - Complete pending blood tests to rule out underlying conditions contributing to fatigue and insomnia.
6. **Health Education:**
   - Educate about the nature of anxiety disorders and their chronic but manageable course.

## SAFETY NETTING:

- Advise to seek urgent care if:
  - Symptoms worsen significantly or new concerning symptoms develop.
  - Experiences thoughts of self-harm or harm to others.

## QUESTIONS:

1. **What is the role of GAD-7 in diagnosis and management of anxiety?**
   - GAD-7 is a validated tool to screen and assess the severity of generalized anxiety disorder. Scores guide initial diagnosis and monitor treatment response.
2. **When should medication be initiated for anxiety?**
   - Medication should be considered in moderate to severe cases or when symptoms are significantly impairing daily functioning and non-pharmacological measures alone are insufficient.
3. **What lifestyle measures can help with anxiety?**
   - Regular exercise, balanced diet, sleep hygiene, reduced caffeine and alcohol, and relaxation techniques are essential.

# CASE 48 Suicidal Ideation

## Doctor's Notes

*Patient Details:*

- **Name:** Sara Ahmed
- **Age:** 14 years
- **Gender:** Female
- **Occupation:** Student
- **Presenting Complaint:** Persistent sadness and suicidal thoughts
- **Setting:** Family Medicine Clinic

## PATIENT'S SIMULATED SCRIPT:

### Opening Statement:

"I don't feel like doing anything anymore, and sometimes I feel like everyone would be better off without me."

## HISTORY:

- **History of Present Illness:**
  - Persistent low mood for the past 3 months, worsening over the past 2 weeks.
  - Loss of interest in previously enjoyed activities like drawing and spending time with friends.
  - Poor concentration affecting academic performance.
  - Fatigue, even after sufficient sleep.
  - Reports feeling worthless and guilt over minor mistakes.
  - Episodes of crying without clear triggers.
  - Appetite decreased, resulting in mild weight loss.
  - Sleep disturbances: Difficulty falling asleep, frequent awakenings, and early morning wakening.
  - Suicidal thoughts: "I think about what it would be like not to exist anymore, but I haven't done anything to hurt myself."

- **Triggers:**
  - Academic stress and difficulty fitting in at school.
  - Recent argument with her best friend, worsening feelings of isolation.
- **Past Medical History:**
  - No known medical or psychiatric illnesses.
- **Family History:**
  - Mother diagnosed with depression, on treatment.
  - Father: Hypertension.
  - No family history of suicide.
- **Drug History:**
  - No regular medications.
  - No known allergies.
- **Social History:**
  - Lives with her parents and two younger siblings.
  - Supportive family but feels misunderstood.
  - No history of substance use.
- **Lifestyle:**
  - Does not exercise regularly.
  - Withdrawn from social activities.

## IDEAS, CONCERNS, EXPECTATIONS:

- **Ideas:** She thinks maybe she is low on vitamins or there's a hormone issue causing her to feel this way.
- **Concerns:** Worried that she won't feel better and that her thoughts may worsen and she'll continue feeling this way.
- **Expectations:** Hopes for a safe space to express herself and a solution to help her feel normal again.

## ON EXAMINATION:

- **General Appearance:** Low eye contact, flat affect, appears tired.
- **Vital Signs:**
  - BP: 108/70 mmHg
  - HR: 72 bpm
  - Temp: 36.7°C
  - $SpO_2$: 98% on room air
- **Mental State Examination:**
  - **Appearance:** Well-groomed but disengaged.
  - **Speech:** Soft and slow.
  - **Mood:** Subjectively and objectively low.
  - **Thought Process:** Logical but preoccupied with feelings of worthlessness.
  - **Suicidal Ideation:** Passive thoughts without intent or plan.
  - **Cognition:** Intact, though attention and concentration are reduced.
  - **Insight and Judgment:** Acknowledges the problem and is willing to seek help.

## INVESTIGATIONS:

1. **PHQ-9 Score:** 21 (severe depression).
2. **CBC:** normal.
3. **TSH and T4:** normal.
4. **Vitamin D:** normal.

## WHAT IS THE DIAGNOSIS?

**Major Depressive Disorder with Suicidal Ideation.**

## OUTLINE THE MANAGEMENT PLAN:

*Immediate Steps:*

1. **Ensure Safety:**
   - Assess for risk of self-harm or suicide:
     - Although she has no immediate intent or plan, discuss a safety plan with the patient and her parents, including supervision and removal of harmful objects.
   - Provide emergency contact numbers for mental health crises.
2. **Psychological Support:**
   - Urgent referral to child and adolescent psychiatry for evaluation and therapy.
   - Recommend cognitive-behavioural therapy (CBT) to address negative thought patterns and build coping strategies.
3. **Pharmacological Therapy (if indicated):**
   - Consider starting fluoxetine (SSRI), starting at 10 mg daily, after psychiatric consultation, as it is FDA-approved for adolescents.

*Address Contributing Factors:*

4. **Family Support:**
   - Involve parents in the treatment plan, with their consent, to ensure a supportive environment.
   - Educate parents about depression and its impact on adolescents.
5. **Lifestyle Modifications:**
   - Encourage regular physical activity to boost mood (e.g., walking, cycling).
   - Promote healthy sleep hygiene practices.
   - Suggest a balanced diet and monitor for nutritional deficiencies.

## FOLLOW-UP:

- Schedule a follow-up visit in 1–2 weeks to monitor symptoms, response to interventions, and safety.
- Monitor for side effects if medication is initiated.

## SAFETY NETTING:

- Advise parents to watch for signs of worsening depression, including:
  - Increased withdrawal.
  - Changes in appetite or sleep patterns.
  - Escalation of suicidal thoughts.

## QUESTIONS:

1. **What are the differential diagnoses for depression in adolescents?**
   - Hypothyroidism.
   - Anaemia.
   - Chronic fatigue syndrome.
   - Adjustment disorder.
   - Bipolar disorder.

2. **What are the key components of a safety plan?**
   - Identifying triggers and warning signs.
   - Providing emergency contact numbers.
   - Establishing coping strategies and supportive contacts.
3. **What lifestyle measures can help manage depression?**
   - Regular exercise.
   - Healthy diet and sleep habits.
   - Stress reduction techniques, such as mindfulness or journaling.

CASE

# Bulimia Nervosa 49

## Doctor's Notes

*Patient Details:*

- **Name:** Layla Hassan
- **Age:** 29 years
- **Gender:** Female
- **Occupation:** Marketing Specialist
- **Presenting Complaint:** Request for weight-loss medication (Mounjaro [tirzepatide])
- **Setting:** Family Medicine Clinic

## PATIENT'S SIMULATED SCRIPT:

### Opening Statement:

"I've heard about Mounjaro for weight loss, and I think it might help me."

## HISTORY:

- **History of Presenting Complaint:**
  - Reports feeling overweight despite a BMI of 23 (normal weight range).
  - Claims to have gained 2 kg in the past 2 weeks.
  - Strong focus on her appearance and fear of further weight gain.
  - Admits to frequent episodes of overeating, often followed by feelings of guilt.
  - Reports inducing vomiting "occasionally" to "stay in control."
- **Associated Symptoms:**
  - Frequent sore throat and dental sensitivity.
  - No history of fainting, significant weight loss, or major dietary changes.
- **Past Medical History:**
  - No chronic illnesses.
  - No previous hospitalizations or surgeries.

- **Drug History:**
  - Multivitamin occasionally.
  - No regular medications.
  - No known drug allergies.
- **Family History:**
  - Mother has type 2 diabetes.
  - Sister with history of anxiety disorder.
- **Lifestyle History:**
  - Non-smoker, occasional alcohol use.
  - Exercises regularly but describes "obsessive" tendencies, such as exercising after meals to "burn calories."
- **Social History:**
  - Lives alone, feels socially pressured about her appearance due to her job in marketing.

## IDEAS, CONCERNS, EXPECTATIONS:

- **Ideas:** Believes weight-loss medications will solve her "weight problem."
- **Concerns:** Worried that she's losing control over her weight.
- **Expectations:** Hopes for a quick and effective solution to her perceived weight gain.

## ON EXAMINATION:

- **General Appearance:** Well-groomed but anxious.
- **Vital Signs:**
  - BP: 110/72 mmHg
  - HR: 72 bpm
  - Temp: 36.5°C
  - BMI: 23 (Normal range)
- **Physical Examination Findings:**
  - Dental erosion visible, suggestive of repeated exposure to stomach acid.
  - Russell sign: Calluses on the knuckles from inducing vomiting.
  - No signs of dehydration or significant malnutrition.

## INVESTIGATIONS:

1. **CBC:** normal
2. **Electrolytes:** normal
3. **Thyroid Panel:** normal
4. **ECG:** normal

## WHAT IS THE DIAGNOSIS?

1. **Bulimia Nervosa** – Recurrent episodes of binge eating followed by compensatory behaviours such as vomiting.
2. **Body Dysmorphic Disorder (possible)** – Preoccupation with perceived weight gain despite a normal BMI.

Bulimia nervosa is a serious eating disorder characterized by a cycle of binge eating – consuming large amounts of food in a short period – followed by behaviours to prevent weight gain, such as self-induced vomiting, misuse of laxatives, fasting, or excessive exercise. Individuals with bulimia often feel a loss of control during binge episodes and may experience feelings of shame or guilt afterward.

## OUTLINE THE MANAGEMENT PLAN:

*Immediate Steps:*

1. **Address Eating Disorder:**
   - Refer to a psychologist or psychiatrist specializing in eating disorders.
   - Initiate cognitive-behavioural therapy (CBT) to address distorted body image and unhealthy eating behaviours.
2. **Pharmacological Therapy:**
   - Consider fluoxetine (SSRI), starting at 20 mg once daily, as it is FDA-approved for bulimia nervosa.
   - Monitor for side effects and adherence.
3. **Nutritional Counselling:**
   - Refer to a dietitian for tailored meal planning and to rebuild a healthy relationship with food.
4. **Monitoring and Safety:**
   - Regular follow-ups to monitor weight, mental health, and physical complications of bulimia.
   - Address dental health by referring to a dentist for treatment of dental erosion.

*Reassurance and Education:*

- **Weight Loss Medication Discussion:**
  - Explain that Mounjaro (tirzepatide) is not indicated for individuals with a normal BMI.
  - Emphasize that her current weight is within a healthy range, and the focus should be on her overall well-being.

## FOLLOW-UP:

1. **Short-Term:**
   - Follow up in 1–2 weeks to assess mood, eating patterns, and adherence to therapy.
2. **Long-Term:**
   - Regular reviews to monitor progress in therapy and nutritional status.
   - Screen for complications such as electrolyte imbalances, arrhythmias, and gastrointestinal issues.

## QUESTIONS:

1. **What are the long-term complications of bulimia nervosa?**
   - Electrolyte imbalances leading to arrhythmias.
   - Oesophageal tears or gastric rupture.
   - Chronic dehydration and renal damage.
   - Severe dental erosion and gum disease.
2. **Why is fluoxetine used in bulimia nervosa?**
   - It helps reduce binge-eating episodes and improves mood; also it is FDA-approved for reducing binge-purge frequency and for improving mood.
3. **How can family and friends support someone with bulimia nervosa?**
   - Encouraging open conversations and being non-judgmental.
   - Avoiding comments about appearance or weight.
   - Supporting treatment adherence and attending family counselling sessions if needed.
4. **How can family and social support optimize recovery in bulimia nervosa?**
   - Through encouraging a non-judgemental environment, where discussions focus on feelings and not "target weights."
   - Encouraging family members to attend therapy sessions together.
5. **If the patient develops severe hypokalaemia and arrhythmias due to vomiting, how should management be prioritized?**
   - Immediate stabilisation: IV potassium replacement, continuous cardiac monitoring, manage dehydration.
   - Addressing the underlying cause: Hospital admission, psychiatric evaluation, therapy initiation.
   - Long term: correct electrolyte imbalance and monitoring for recurrence.

# CASE 50
# General Anxiety Disorder and Adjustment Disorder

## Doctor's Notes

*Patient Details:*

- **Name:** Omar Khalil
- **Age:** 29 years
- **Gender:** Male
- **Occupation:** First-year medical student
- **Presenting Complaint:** Social withdrawal and difficulty concentrating; later development of excessive worrying and generalized anxiety
- **Setting:** Family Medicine Clinic

## PATIENT'S SIMULATED SCRIPT:

### Opening Statement:

"I feel overwhelmed, and it's getting harder to focus."

## HISTORY:

- **History of Presenting Complaint:**
  - Initially reported social withdrawal and difficulty concentrating during the first semester of medical school.
  - Symptoms progressed over the last 5 months to include excessive worrying about academic performance, relationships, and personal health.
  - Reports feeling tense most of the day and having difficulty falling asleep due to racing thoughts.
  - Complains of fatigue, muscle tension, and irritability.
- **Associated Symptoms:**
  - No panic attacks or specific phobias.
  - No history of traumatic events.
- **Impact on Life:**
  - Grades have declined significantly.
  - Avoids social interactions with classmates and family.
  - Struggles to engage in enjoyable activities due to persistent anxiety.

- **Past Medical History:**
  - No chronic illnesses.
  - No hospitalizations or surgeries.
- **Drug History:**
  - Occasionally takes over-the-counter melatonin for sleep.
  - No regular medications.
  - No known drug allergies.
- **Family History:**
  - Father has a history of depression.
  - Mother has generalized anxiety disorder.
- **Lifestyle and Social History:**
  - Non-smoker, no alcohol or recreational drug use.
  - Eats irregularly due to stress, often skipping meals.
  - Reduced physical activity since starting medical school.

## IDEAS, CONCERNS, EXPECTATIONS:

- **Ideas:** Wonders if his symptoms are due to the stress of medical school.
- **Concerns:** Fears he is not capable of handling the pressure and may fail.
- **Expectations:** Hopes for advice or treatment to help manage his anxiety and regain focus.

## ON EXAMINATION:

- **General Appearance:** Appears tense and fatigued.
- **Vital Signs:**
  - BP: 122/76 mmHg
  - HR: 88 bpm
  - Temp: 36.8°C
- **Mental State Examination:**
  - Alert and oriented.
  - Speech is normal but slightly slow.
  - Mood: Anxious.
  - Thought process: Logical but preoccupied with worries.
  - No hallucinations, delusions, or suicidal ideation.

## INVESTIGATIONS:

- **Generalized Anxiety Disorder Assessment (GAD-7):** Score of 17 (severe anxiety).
- **CBC, TSH, Vitamin $B_{12}$:** Normal, ruling out organic causes of fatigue and poor concentration.

## WHAT IS THE DIAGNOSIS?

1. **Generalized Anxiety Disorder (GAD)** – Persistent excessive worry affecting daily functioning.
2. **Adjustment Disorder with Depressed Mood (initial presentation)** – Social withdrawal and concentration difficulties likely triggered by medical school stress.

## MANAGEMENT PLAN

*Immediate Steps:*

1. **Psychological Therapy:**
    - Refer for cognitive behavioural therapy (CBT) to address cognitive distortions and develop coping strategies.
    - Encourage mindfulness-based stress reduction techniques.
2. **Pharmacological Therapy:**
    - Initiate escitalopram (SSRI) 10 mg once daily, with plans to reassess in 2–4 weeks.
    - Consider hydroxyzine as needed for acute anxiety episodes.
3. **Lifestyle Modifications:**
    - Establish a regular sleep schedule and promote sleep hygiene.
    - Encourage a balanced diet with regular meals.
    - Recommend moderate-intensity exercise (e.g., brisk walking or yoga) for at least 30 minutes, 5 days a week.
4. **Social Support:**
    - Suggest joining a peer support group for medical students.
    - Encourage reconnecting with family and friends for emotional support.

*Reassurance and Education:*

- Explain that anxiety disorders are common and highly treatable.
- Emphasize the importance of early intervention to prevent worsening symptoms.

## FOLLOW-UP:

1. **Short-Term:**
    - Weekly or biweekly follow-ups to monitor medication side effects, therapy progress, and symptom changes.
2. **Long-Term:**
    - Regular reviews every 1–3 months to adjust treatment as needed.

## QUESTIONS:

1. **What are the differential diagnoses for persistent worry and difficulty concentrating?**
    - Generalized Anxiety Disorder (GAD).
    - Adjustment Disorder.
    - Major Depressive Disorder (MDD).
    - Attention Deficit–Hyperactivity Disorder (ADHD).
2. **What are the side effects of escitalopram?**
    - Nausea, dry mouth, drowsiness, or insomnia.
    - Potential sexual side effects.
3. **What are the long-term goals of GAD treatment?**
    - Reduction in anxiety symptoms.
    - Improved functioning in academic, social, and personal life.
    - Development of effective coping mechanisms.

CASE 51

# Premenstrual Dysphoric Disorder

## Doctor's Notes

*Patient Details:*

- **Name:** Haya Ali
- **Age:** 32 years
- **Gender:** Female
- **Occupation:** Marketing Manager
- **Presenting Complaint:** Emotional and physical symptoms prior to menstruation affecting her daily functioning
- **Setting:** Family Medicine Clinic

## PATIENT'S SIMULATED SCRIPT:

### Opening Statement:

"I feel like I'm a completely different person before my period starts."

## HISTORY:

- **History of Presenting Complaint:**
  - Reports irritability, mood swings, anxiety, and depression beginning 7–10 days before menstruation and resolving shortly after her period starts.
  - Associated physical symptoms include breast tenderness, bloating, and fatigue.
  - Symptoms have been ongoing for over a year and significantly affect her work and relationships.
- **Impact on Life:**
  - Difficulty concentrating at work and frequent conflicts with colleagues and family during symptomatic days.
- **Past Medical History:**
  - Mild anxiety managed previously with counselling; no history of major depression or psychiatric hospitalizations.
  - No chronic medical conditions.
- **Drug History:**
  - Occasionally takes over-the-counter pain medication for menstrual cramps.
  - No regular medications.
  - No known drug allergies.

- **Family History:**
  - Mother experienced similar symptoms before menopause.
  - Father has type 2 diabetes.
- **Lifestyle and Social History:**
  - Non-smoker, no alcohol or recreational drug use.
  - Irregular exercise due to fatigue.
  - Balanced diet but craves sweets and salty snacks during the symptomatic phase.

## IDEAS, CONCERNS, EXPECTATIONS:

- **Ideas:** Wonders if her hormones are out of balance.
- **Concerns:** Worries that her symptoms might worsen with age or lead to depression.
- **Expectations:** Hopes for treatment to improve her quality of life and manage her emotional and physical symptoms.

## ON EXAMINATION:

- **General Appearance:** Appears well but looks mildly fatigued.
- **Vital Signs:**
  - BP: 116/74 mmHg
  - HR: 76 bpm
  - Temp: 36.7°C
- **Mental State Examination:**
  - Alert and oriented.
  - Mood: Euthymic today, but reports mood changes before menstruation.
  - Thought process: Logical, no suicidal ideation.

## INVESTIGATIONS:

1. **Prospective Symptom Diary:** Recommended tracking symptoms for two to three menstrual cycles to confirm timing and severity.
2. **Hormonal Tests:** Normal (to rule out thyroid or other endocrine disorders).
3. **Psychological Assessment:** GAD-7 and PHQ-9 are normal, supporting PMDD rather than a primary mood disorder.

## WHAT IS THE DIAGNOSIS?

**Premenstrual Dysphoric Disorder (PMDD)** – Severe affective and physical symptoms in the luteal phase of the menstrual cycle.

PMDD is a severe form of premenstrual syndrome (PMS) that significantly affects a person's emotional and physical well-being in the days leading up to menstruation. Unlike typical PMS, PMDD causes intense mood swings, irritability, depression, and anxiety, which can interfere with daily life and relationships.

## OUTLINE THE MANAGEMENT PLAN:

*Immediate Steps:*

1. **Lifestyle Modifications:**
   - Encourage regular aerobic exercise (30 minutes, 5 times a week) to reduce symptoms.
   - Advise a balanced diet, limiting caffeine, alcohol, and refined sugars.
   - Promote adequate sleep hygiene.

2. **Psychological Interventions:**
   - Refer for cognitive behavioural therapy (CBT) to help manage mood symptoms.
3. **Pharmacological Therapy:**
   - Start sertraline (SSRI) at a low dose of 50 mg once daily, titrate based on response.
   - Discuss side effects, including potential gastrointestinal symptoms or insomnia.
4. **Supplementation:**
   - Recommend calcium carbonate (1200 mg daily) to alleviate physical symptoms.
   - Vitamin $B_6$ (50–100 mg daily) may help with mood symptoms.
5. **Follow-up Plan:**
   - Review in 4–6 weeks to assess response to treatment and adjust therapy if needed.

## SAFETY NETTING:

- Advise to return if symptoms worsen or if she develops any thoughts of self-harm or harm to others.
- Provide reassurance that PMDD is a treatable condition.

## QUESTIONS:

1. **What are the differential diagnoses for premenstrual dysphoric disorder?**
   - **Premenstrual Syndrome (PMS):** Less severe emotional and physical symptoms without significant functional impairment.
   - **Major Depressive Disorder (MDD):** Persistent low mood and other symptoms not restricted to the luteal phase.
   - **Generalized Anxiety Disorder (GAD):** Chronic excessive worry unrelated to the menstrual cycle.
   - **Thyroid Dysfunction:** Symptoms such as fatigue or mood changes may mimic PMDD.
2. **How do you manage discontinuation syndrome from stopping an SSRI abruptly?**
   - Gradually taper the dose over 2–4 weeks (or longer, depending on the duration of use).
   - Address withdrawal symptoms (e.g., dizziness, irritability, flu-like symptoms) with reassurance and symptomatic treatment.
   - If severe symptoms occur, consider reinstating the SSRI and tapering more slowly.
3. **If symptoms do not respond to SSRIs or lifestyle measures, what is the next step in management?**
   - **GnRH agonists (e.g., leuprolide):** Induce temporary ovarian suppression for severe, refractory cases.
   - **Combined oral contraceptives:** Certain formulations (e.g., drospirenone/ethinyl estradiol) can stabilize hormonal fluctuations.
4. **What is the evidence for calcium and vitamin B6 in the management of this condition?**
   - Calcium at 1200 mg daily aids in neuromuscular stabilisation, which reduces physical and affective symptoms.
   - Vitamin $B_6$ at 50- to 100-mg dose daily improves mood symptoms via neurotransmitter synthesis.
   - The above are both safe medications to consider prescribing alongside SSRs.

# CASE 52 Hernia

## Doctor's Notes

*Patient Details:*

- **Name:** Ahmed Salim
- **Age:** 22 years
- **Gender:** Male
- **Occupation:** University student
- **Presenting Complaint:** Pain and swelling in the right groin
- **Setting:** Family Medicine Clinic

## PATIENT'S SIMULATED SCRIPT:

### Opening Statement:

"I have this painful lump in my groin that's not going away."

## HISTORY:

- **History of Presenting Complaint:**
  - Lump in the right groin noticed 2 days ago, initially reducible but became painful and irreducible yesterday.
  - Associated symptoms: Swelling, redness, and tenderness in the groin area.
  - No fever, vomiting, or change in bowel habits.
- **Past Medical History:**
  - No previous hernia repairs.
  - No known chronic conditions or surgeries.
- **Drug History:**
  - No regular medications.
  - No known allergies.
- **Family History:**
  - Father had a history of inguinal hernia surgery.

- **Lifestyle and Social History:**
  - Non-smoker.
  - Exercises regularly, including weightlifting.
  - Balanced diet.

## IDEAS, CONCERNS, EXPECTATIONS:

- **Ideas:** Thinks he might have an infection.
- **Concerns:** Worried that the pain may get worse.
- **Expectations:** Seeks a solution to relieve the pain and swelling and prevent recurrence.

## EXAMINATION:

- **General Appearance:** Mild discomfort but alert and oriented.
- **Vital Signs:**
  - BP: 120/80 mmHg
  - HR: 88 bpm
  - Temp: 36.8°C
  - $SpO_2$: 98% on room air
- **Inspection:**
  - Visible swelling in the right groin, erythematous skin overlying the lump.
  - Lump is tense and irreducible.
- **Palpation:**
  - Tender, firm mass in the right inguinal region.
  - Positive cough impulse absent.
  - No bowel sounds auscultated over the lump.
- **Abdominal Examination:**
  - Soft, non-tender.
  - No distension or masses.

## INVESTIGATIONS:

1. **Bedside Ultrasound (if requested):**
   - Confirms incarcerated inguinal hernia with no signs of strangulation.
2. **Blood Tests (if ordered):**
   - **WBC:** Normal
   - **CRP:** Normal
   - **Electrolytes:** Normal

## WHAT IS THE DIAGNOSIS?

**Incarcerated Inguinal Hernia.**

An incarcerated inguinal hernia occurs when a portion of tissue, such as the intestine, protrudes through a weak spot in the lower abdominal wall into the groin area and becomes trapped. This entrapment prevents the tissue from moving back into the abdomen, leading to a painful bulge in the groin. If left untreated, it can cut off blood flow to the trapped intestine, leading to tissue death, a life-threatening condition requiring immediate surgery.

## OUTLINE THE MANAGEMENT PLAN:

*Immediate Steps:*

1. **Referral to General Surgery:**
   - Urgent referral for surgical assessment and repair.
   - Educate the patient about the risks of delaying treatment (e.g., strangulation, bowel ischaemia).
2. **Pain Management:**
   - Prescribe paracetamol 1 g every 6 hours as needed.
   - Avoid NSAIDs until surgical evaluation due to potential bleeding risks.
3. **Lifestyle Advice:**
   - Advise against lifting heavy weights or straining, to avoid further hernias developing.

*Long-Term Management:*

1. **After Surgery:**
   - Wound care and follow-up to ensure proper healing.
   - Encourage weight management and safe lifting techniques to reduce recurrence risk.

## QUESTIONS:

1. **What are the differential diagnoses for a groin lump?**
   - Inguinal or femoral hernia (direct or indirect).
   - Lymphadenopathy.
   - Testicular torsion or hydrocele.
   - Lipoma or abscess.
2. **What are the complications of an incarcerated hernia if untreated?**
   - Strangulation, leading to bowel ischaemia and necrosis.
   - Intestinal obstruction.
3. **How does one clinically distinguish between an incarcerated and a strangulated hernia?**
   - Incarcerated = Irreducible lump, tender, often without systemic signs. In this kind of hernia, the bowel is still viable.
   - Irreducible + severe pain, skin changes (dusky, purple), systemic toxicity (tachycardia, fever, leucocytosis, acidosis), absent bowel sounds, peritonitis possible. In this kind of hernia, the bowel may be necrosed/dead or dying.
4. **When is imaging indicated in a suspected groin hernia, and which modality is preferred?**
   - Diagnosed clinically; however, if there is uncertainty, ultrasound is helpful in distinguishing between hernias, lymph nodes, or abscesses.
   - CT scan: If the diagnosis is still unclear and there is a need to differentiate between inguinal versus femoral hernias, typically when managing obese patients.
5. **What are common risk factors for inguinal hernia development in young adults?**
   - Congenital – indirect hernias (patent processus vaginalis)
   - Acquired – heavy lifting, chronic cough, constipation
   - Family history
   - Male gender
   - Connective tissue disorders such as Ehler–Danlos and Marfan syndrome

CASE

# Compartment Syndrome 53

## Doctor's Notes

*Patient Details:*

- **Name:** Khalid Ahmed
- **Age:** 45 years
- **Gender:** Male
- **Occupation:** Businessman
- **Presenting Complaint:** Left lower leg pain following a motorbike collision
- **Setting:** Family Medicine Clinic

## PATIENT'S SIMULATED SCRIPT (INITIAL VISIT):

### Opening Statement:

"I was hit by a motorbike delivery guy, and my leg hurts a lot."

## HISTORY:

- **History of Presenting Complaint:**
  - Incident occurred 3 hours ago when a delivery rider struck his left leg.
  - Complains of localized pain and swelling in the lower leg.
  - Able to bear weight but with discomfort.
  - No numbness, tingling, or weakness initially.
- **Past Medical History:**
  - No chronic illnesses.
  - No previous fractures or surgeries.
- **Drug History:**
  - No regular medications.
  - No known allergies.

- **Lifestyle and Social History:**
  - Non-smoker, no alcohol consumption.
  - Sedentary work but walks regularly for exercise.
- **Family History:**
  - No relevant conditions.

## EXAMINATION:

*Vital Signs:*

- BP: 128/80 mmHg
- HR: 86 bpm
- Temp: 36.7°C
- $SpO_2$: 99% on room air

*Left Leg Examination:*

- Swelling and tenderness over the mid-lower leg.
- No deformity or open wounds.
- Intact skin with normal distal pulses.
- No paraesthesia or weakness on neurological examination.

## INVESTIGATIONS:

- **X-ray (initial visit):**
  - Non-displaced fracture of the midshaft of the fibula.
  - No signs of dislocation or additional fractures.

## DIAGNOSIS:

**Non-Displaced Midshaft Fibula Fracture.**

## MANAGEMENT:

*Initial Visit*

1. **Immobilization and Pain Management:**
   - Apply a below-knee splint.
   - Prescribe paracetamol 1 g every 6 hours as needed for pain.
2. **Activity Modification:**
   - Advise rest, elevation of the leg, and avoidance of weight-bearing.
   - Use crutches if necessary.
3. **Follow-up Instructions:**
   - Schedule a review in 1 week to assess healing and symptoms.
4. **Safety Netting:**
   - Advise to return immediately if numbness, increased pain, or change in sensation develops.

## FOLLOW-UP VISIT:

### Opening Statement:

"I've been feeling more pain and numbness in my leg since last night."

## UPDATED HISTORY:

- **Symptoms:**
  - Worsening pain in the left leg over the past 24 hours, unrelieved by medication.
  - Numbness and tingling sensation in the lower leg.
  - Feeling of tightness in the leg.
  - No fever, chills, or discharge from the splint site.

## UPDATED EXAMINATION:

*General Appearance:*
- Appears in significant discomfort.

*Left Leg Examination:*
- Severe swelling and tension in the lower leg.
- Skin is taut and shiny.
- Pain on passive stretching of the toes.
- Decreased sensation over the dorsum of the foot.
- Capillary refill is slightly delayed, and dorsalis pedis pulse is faint.

## WHAT IS THE DIAGNOSIS?

**Compartment Syndrome** secondary to fibula fracture.

Compartment syndrome is a serious condition where increased pressure within a confined space in the body, usually a muscle compartment, restricts blood flow to the tissues within that space.

This lack of blood flow can lead to tissue damage and, if not treated promptly, permanent injury. It often occurs after severe injuries, such as fractures or crush injuries, and commonly affects the legs but can also occur in the arms, hands, feet, and buttocks.

## OUTLINE THE MANAGEMENT PLAN:

1. **Immediate Steps:**
   - **Urgent Referral to Orthopaedics:** Emergency fasciotomy to relieve compartment pressure.
   - **Pain Management:** Administer intravenous morphine for severe pain.
   - **Monitoring:** Closely monitor neurovascular status of the affected leg during transfer.
2. **Long-Term Management:**
   - After fasciotomy:
     - Monitor for infection and wound healing.
     - Ensure proper fracture care, including immobilization and rehabilitation.
3. **Education:**
   - Explain the risk of compartment syndrome to the patient and emphasize early reporting of symptoms in the future.

## QUESTIONS:

1. **What are the signs of compartment syndrome?**
   - Severe pain, especially on passive stretch.
   - Swelling, tightness, and shiny appearance of the skin.
   - Numbness or tingling in the affected area.
   - Weak or absent distal pulses (late sign).

2. **How is compartment syndrome treated?**
   - Emergency fasciotomy to release pressure and prevent permanent damage to muscles and nerves.
3. **What is the pathophysiology of compartment syndrome?**
   - There is increased intracompartmental pressure exceeding capillary perfusion pressure and reduced tissue perfusion, which results in ischaemia and muscle necrosis.
4. **Can you outline the 6 Ps of compartment syndrome?**
   - Pain
   - Pallor
   - Paraesthesia
   - Paralysis
   - Pulselessness
   - Poikilothermia (cold limb)

# CASE 54 Gallstones

## Doctor's Notes

*Patient Details:*

- **Name:** Mahmoud Al-Ansari
- **Age:** 50 years
- **Gender:** Male
- **Occupation:** Shop owner
- **Presenting Complaint:** Stomach pain
- **Setting:** Family Medicine Clinic

## PATIENT'S SIMULATED SCRIPT:

### Opening Statement:

"I've been having stomach pain and feeling feverish."

## HISTORY:

- **History of Presenting Complaint:**
  - Pain started 2 days ago, located in the upper right side of the abdomen, radiating to the back.
  - Associated with nausea, vomiting, and intermittent fever with chills.
  - Reports yellowish discoloration of the eyes starting yesterday.
  - No significant change in bowel habits or urine colour.
- **Past Medical History:**
  - Known gallstones diagnosed 1 year ago, no prior interventions.
  - Hypertension for 5 years, controlled on amlodipine.
- **Drug History:**
  - Amlodipine 10 mg daily.
  - No known drug allergies.
- **Family History:**
  - Mother had gallbladder disease.
  - Father passed away from a stroke at 70.

- **Lifestyle and Social History:**
  - Smoker: 1 pack/day for 25 years.
  - Occasional alcohol use.
  - Sedentary lifestyle and a high-fat diet.

## IDEAS, CONCERNS, EXPECTATIONS:

- **Ideas:** Patient is unsure what might be causing the pain but feels it could be serious.
- **Concerns:** Worried about the fever and yellowing of the eyes.
- **Expectations:** Hopes to get relief from the pain and a clear explanation of what is happening.

## EXAMINATION:

- **General Appearance:**
  - Ill-appearing, febrile, and mildly jaundiced.
- **Vital Signs:**
  - Temperature: 38.7°C
  - BP: 130/85 mmHg
  - HR: 104 bpm, regular
  - $SpO_2$: 97% on room air
- **Abdominal Examination:**
  - Tenderness in the right upper quadrant (RUQ) with guarding.
  - Positive Murphy sign.
  - No palpable masses or organomegaly.
- **Other Findings:**
  - Mild scleral icterus.
  - No evidence of peripheral oedema or signs of chronic liver disease.

## WHAT IS THE DIAGNOSIS?

**Acute Cholangitis.**

Gallstones form when bile, a fluid made by the liver to help digest fats, turns into solid stones. These stones are often made of hardened fatty substances, like cholesterol. Sometimes they consist of bile pigments (a substance that gives bile its colour) or calcium deposits. There might be just a few small stones, a lot of tiny stones, or one large stone.

## OUTLINE THE MANAGEMENT PLAN:

*Immediate Steps:*

1. **Urgent Referral:**
   - Refer to the emergency department for inpatient management and further evaluation.
2. **Supportive Care:**
   - NPO (nothing by mouth) to rest the gastrointestinal system.
   - Intravenous fluids to maintain hydration and haemodynamic stability.
   - Administer antipyretics (e.g., paracetamol) to manage fever.
3. **Empiric Antibiotics:**
   - Start broad-spectrum antibiotics targeting gram-negative and anaerobic bacteria (e.g., IV piperacillin-tazobactam or ceftriaxone with metronidazole).

## QUESTIONS:

1. **What are your top four differential diagnoses?**
   - Acute cholecystitis
   - Hepatitis (viral or alcoholic)
   - Pancreatitis
   - Peptic ulcer disease
2. **What signs do you look for?**
   - **Charcot Triad:** RUQ pain, fever, and jaundice (suggestive of cholangitis).
   - **Reynold Pentad:** Charcot triad + hypotension and altered mental status (indicating severe cholangitis).
3. **What investigations should you consider in a case of suspected cholangitis?**
   - **Blood Tests:** CBC, liver function tests, serum bilirubin, amylase/lipase, and blood cultures.
   - **Imaging:** Abdominal ultrasound (to identify biliary dilatation or stones).
   - **Further Imaging:** Magnetic resonance cholangiopancreatography (MRCP) if ultrasound findings are inconclusive.
4. **What is the mechanism that causes acute cholangitis?**
   - Blockage of the common bile duct by gallstones, resulting in bile stasis and bacterial overgrowth, leading to ascending infection and sepsis.
5. **What is the gold standard definitive treatment?**
   - ERCP (decompresses the biliary tree) and stent insertion afterwards.

# CASE 55
# Telogen Effluvium

## Doctor's Notes

***Patient Details:***

- **Name:** Daina Sam
- **Age:** 21 years
- **Ethnicity:** Caucasian
- **Gender:** Female
- **Occupation:** Second-year college student (Aerospace Engineering)
- **Presenting Complaint:** Hair loss
- **Setting:** Family Medicine Clinic

## PATIENT'S SIMULATED SCRIPT:

### Background:

A second-year college student visiting the Family Medicine Clinic during a break after stressful final exams. She has been living in a dormitory since her freshman year and visits her family three times a year, enjoying home-cooked meals when she does.

### Opening Statement:

"Doctor, I've been losing so much hair, and my hair has been looking thinner than usual."

## HISTORY OF PRESENTING COMPLAINT:

- **Site:** Scalp, predominantly thinning at the temples/sides.
- **Onset:** Started 3 months ago.
- **Duration:** Continuous, most noticeable during showering and brushing.
- **Progression:** Worsening, with small clumps of hair now shedding during washing.
- **Aggravating Factors:** Increased shedding during exam season.
- **Relieving Factors:** None attempted.

- **Associated Symptoms:**
  - **Positive:** Brittle nails that break easily and are difficult to grow.
  - **Negative:** No scalp itching, redness, scaling, brittle hair, loss of eyebrows or eyelashes, skin changes (bruising, rashes, stretch marks), fever, or recent weight loss (except for a 10 kg loss during freshman year, which has since stabilized). No visual disturbances, galactorrhoea, or systemic symptoms.

## MEDICAL HISTORY:

- **Past Medical History:** No chronic illnesses.
- **Medication History:** No current medications.
- **Family History:**
  - Sister (25 years old) has Hashimoto thyroiditis, well-controlled.
  - No family history of hair loss.
- **Social History:**
  - **Lifestyle:** Introverted, enjoys studying and working on projects.
  - **Diet:** Limited protein intake, mostly bread, cheese, and tea. Usually eats a snack bar for lunch and a vegetarian wrap if available. Rarely eats fresh fruits or vegetables.
  - **Exercise:** Walks to classes but has no structured workout routine.
  - **Habits:** Non-smoker, does not consume alcohol.
- **Menstrual History:**
  - Irregular cycles (approximately every 3 months).
  - Heavy flow with occasional clots; manages cramps with heating pads.
- **Obstetric and Gynaecological History:**
  - Not sexually active, has never been pregnant.

## IDEAS, CONCERNS, EXPECTATIONS:

- **Ideas:** Worried that hair loss could be genetic or linked to an underlying health condition.
- **Concerns:** Feels frustrated and less confident compared to family members and peers.
- **Expectations:** Wants to identify the cause and restore hair health.

## EXAMINATION FINDINGS:

- **General:** Healthy appearance, no pallor, jaundice, or systemic illness.
- **Hair:**
  - Diffuse thinning, more prominent at the temples and sides.
  - Positive hair pull test (>10% hair shed).
  - No redness, scarring, or scaling.
- **Skin and Nails:**
  - Brittle nails, prone to breaking.
  - No bruising, stretch marks, or lesions.
- **Systemic Examination:** Normal.
- **Thyroid Examination:** Normal.

## PRIMARY DIAGNOSIS:

**Telogen Effluvium.**

Telogen effluvium is a common condition where the individual experiences noticeable hair shedding, often seeing more hair than usual in the hairbrush, shower, or on the pillow. This happens because the body's natural hair growth cycle is temporarily disrupted, causing more hairs to enter the shedding phase simultaneously. Common triggers include significant stress, major life events, illness, or drastic changes in diet. Telogen effluvium is typically temporary.

## OUTLINE THE MANAGEMENT PLAN:

**What baseline bloods are important to consider testing for in a case of suspected telogen effluvium?**

- Complete blood count (CBC).
- Ferritin and iron studies (TIBC).
- Thyroid function tests (TSH, free T4, free T3).
- Vitamin D, $B_{12}$, zinc levels.
- Hormonal profile (LH, FSH, testosterone) if PCOS is suspected.

**Patient Education and Reassurance:**

- Explain that telogen effluvium is usually **temporary and reversible.**
- Discuss the role of stress and diet in hair loss.
- Recommend **stress management techniques** (e.g., relaxation exercises, mindfulness).

**Dietary and Lifestyle Modifications:**

- Encourage a balanced diet rich in protein, iron, and vitamins (e.g., legumes, leafy greens, fortified cereals).
- Increase protein intake with easy-to-prepare sources (e.g., nuts, dairy, eggs if acceptable).
- Light exercise to improve overall health.

**Supplementation:**

- Iron supplements if iron deficiency is confirmed.
- Multivitamins with biotin to support hair and nail health.

## FOLLOW-UP:

- Review in 4–6 weeks to assess progression and discuss investigation results.
- Consider referral to Dermatology if no improvement or signs of scarring alopecia appear.

## QUESTIONS:

1. **What is the typical duration/prognosis of telogen effluvium once the underlying cause has been addressed?**
    - 6–12 months; hair shedding improves as it slows in the first 3–6 months.
    - Full regrowth can take up to 12 months.
2. **What clinical signs would make you consider a diagnosis other than telogen effluvium?**
    - Scarring, scaling, and/or pustules on the scalp.
    - Patchy/band like hair loss.
    - Systemic features: weight changes, galactorrhoea, hirsutism.
    - Rapid progression causing bald patches.

# CASE 56 Varicose Veins

## Doctor's Notes

*Patient Details:*

- **Name:** Sarah Ahmed
- **Age:** 45 years
- **Gender:** Female
- **Occupation:** Office Worker
- **Presenting Complaint:** Leg discomfort and bulging veins
- **Setting:** Family Medicine Clinic

## PATIENT'S SIMULATED SCRIPT:

### Opening Statement:

"I've been noticing discomfort in my legs, and these bulging veins just seem to keep getting worse."

## HISTORY:

- **History of Presenting Complaint:**
  - Reports a dull ache and heaviness in her legs, worsening by the end of the day.
  - Discomfort is exacerbated by prolonged sitting at her desk job.
  - Symptoms improve with leg elevation at home.
  - Over the past few months, she has noticed prominent, slightly itchy veins along the inner legs.
- **Past Medical History:**
  - No prior diagnosis of venous disease.
  - No history of deep vein thrombosis (DVT) or leg ulcers.
- **Drug History:**
  - Occasionally takes paracetamol for leg pain.
  - No known drug allergies.
- **Family History:**
  - Mother had leg pain but no confirmed diagnosis.
  - No family history of clotting disorders.

- **Lifestyle and Social History:**
  - Non-smoker, occasional alcohol use.
  - Sedentary lifestyle due to her desk job.
  - Lives with her husband and two teenage children.

## IDEAS, CONCERNS, EXPECTATIONS:

- **Ideas:** Suspects her symptoms might be due to poor circulation from sitting for long hours.
- **Concerns:** Fears the veins might worsen or lead to complications like blood clots.
- **Expectations:** Hopes to learn about non-surgical management options and lifestyle changes.

## EXAMINATION:

- **General Appearance:**
  - Well-appearing, no acute distress.
- **Vital Signs:**
  - Temperature: 36.8°C
  - BP: 125/80 mmHg
  - HR: 78 bpm, regular
  - $SpO_2$: 98% on room air
- **Lower Limb Examination:**
  - Visible twisted and distended veins along the inner lower legs.
  - Mild skin discolouration around the ankles.
  - No evidence of ulcers, oedema, or signs of DVT.
  - Pulses palpable and normal bilaterally.

## WHAT IS THE DIAGNOSIS?

**Varicose Veins** secondary to chronic venous insufficiency.

Varicose veins are enlarged, twisted veins that often appear on the legs. They occur because the tiny valves in the veins, which help blood flow back to the heart, stop working properly. When these valves don't close as they should, blood can pool in the veins, making them bulge and twist.

There might be a feeling of heaviness, aching, or discomfort in the legs, especially after standing or sitting for long periods. Some people notice skin changes or mild swelling. They are usually not dangerous and can often be managed with simple lifestyle changes, such as elevating the legs, wearing compression stockings, and staying active.

## OUTLINE THE MANAGEMENT PLAN:

1. **Conservative Approach**
   - Educate on lifestyle modifications:
     - Regular leg elevation during and after work.
     - Increase physical activity, such as walking or cycling.
     - Avoid prolonged sitting or standing.
   - Recommend graduated compression stockings to reduce symptoms.
2. **Symptomatic Relief**
   - Advise NSAIDs (e.g., ibuprofen) for pain management if required.
3. **Referral**
   - Refer to a vascular specialist if symptoms persist or worsen to discuss:
     - Sclerotherapy.
     - Endovenous laser treatment.
     - Surgical options for vein removal.

## FURTHER INVESTIGATIONS:

- **Duplex Ultrasound:** Assess venous reflux and evaluate deeper veins for valve incompetence.
- **Doppler Ultrasound:** Confirm blood flow patterns and rule out other causes.

## FOLLOW-UP AND SAFETY NETTING:

- Review in 4–6 weeks to monitor symptoms and response to conservative measures.
- Advise immediate medical attention if signs of DVT or worsening symptoms develop.

## QUESTIONS:

1. **What are the signs of chronic venous insufficiency?**
   - Varicose veins, oedema, pigmentation (haemosiderin deposition) and sometimes venous ulcers.
2. **When should we consider a duplex ultrasound scan?**
   - When varicoceles are not responding to conservative therapy.
   - When you suspect deep vein involvement or there is an atypical clinical presentation.
   - When you are considering surgical interventions.
3. **What lifestyle advice can help a patient's varicosities from progressing?**
   - Elevating legs 15–20 minutes a day, several times a day.
   - Partaking in regular exercise.
   - Weight reduction.
   - General avoidance of prolonged sitting or standing, taking regular breaks to walk or stretch.

# CASE 57 Hyperhidrosis

## Doctor's Notes

*Patient Details:*

- **Name:** Yousef Beltagi
- **Age:** 16
- **Occupation:** Mechanical engineering student
- **Presenting Complaint:** Excessive sweating
- **Setting:** Family Medicine Clinic

## PATIENT'S SIMULATED SCRIPT:

### Opening Statement:

"Doctor, I've been sweating since I was in third grade, but after puberty it started increasing, and now that I am going to college it's embarrassing and it's affecting my studying."

## HISTORY:

- **Onset:** Symptoms started when at around 9 years of age, progressively worsening after puberty.
- **Frequency:** Daily, regardless of activity or temperature, though worse during stressful situations.
- **Location:** Excessive sweating primarily on palms, soles, and lately underarms.
- **Triggers:** Stress, anxiety, warm weather, and sometimes no apparent reason.
- **Impact:** Affects exams (exam paper becomes damp when holding it); patient avoids shaking hands or wearing certain clothes; affects holding phone or any touch screen. Sometimes affects going out for dinner, holding cutlery and glassware.

## ATTEMPTS TO MANAGE:

- Tried multiple topical treatments at a young age.
- Tried Botox injections after puberty.
- Frequently changes clothes.

## DRUG HISTORY:

- **Regular Medications:** None.
- **Allergies:** None known.
- **Recent Treatments:** None specific for hyperhidrosis.

## FAMILY HISTORY:

- None

## IDEAS, CONCERNS, EXPECTATIONS:

- **Ideas:** Wonders if it could be related to anxiety, stress, or simply that thinking about it is a trigger.
- **Concerns:** Worried it might be a sign of an underlying health issue or a lifelong condition.
- **Expectations:** Looking for effective treatment to control sweating and improve his quality of life.

## ON EXAMINATION:

- **General Appearance:** Well-groomed but appears anxious.
- **Vital Signs:** BP 120/80 mmHg, HR 88 bpm (regular), temperature 36.8°C.
- **Skin Examination:**
  - Palms visibly damp, foot and axillary areas show significant sweat patches.
  - No signs of skin infection or irritation from excessive sweating.
- **Other Systems:** Normal findings; no systemic symptoms suggestive of an underlying condition.

## WHAT IS THE DIAGNOSIS?

**Primary Focal Hyperhidrosis.**

Excessive sweating in specific areas (palms, soles, underarms) without an underlying medical cause, likely due to over-activity of sweat glands regulated by the sympathetic nervous system.

## OUTLINE THE MANAGEMENT OPTIONS:

1. **Conservative Measures:**
   - **Antiperspirants:** Recommend aluminium chloride-based antiperspirants (e.g., Drysol or Driclor), applied at night.
   - **Lifestyle Changes:** Advise loose, breathable clothing and avoidance of triggers such as spicy food, alcohol, and caffeine.
2. **Medical Interventions:**
   - **Topical Treatments:** Glycopyrronium wipes for localized sweating.
   - **Oral Medications:** Low-dose anticholinergic medications (e.g., oxybutynin) if topical treatments are insufficient.
   - **Botox Injections:** Highly effective for severe axillary hyperhidrosis, requiring repeat treatments every 6–9 months.
3. **Advanced Options (if refractory):**
   - **Iontophoresis:** Useful for palmar/plantar hyperhidrosis; involves passing a low electrical current through water on affected areas.
   - **Surgical Intervention:** Endoscopic thoracic sympathectomy considered in extreme, resistant cases.

## FOLLOW-UP AND SAFETY NETTING:

- **Follow-up:**
  - Review response to initial treatment in 4–6 weeks.
  - Refer to Dermatology for surgery or further intervention if no improvement.
- **Red Flags:**
  - New generalized sweating or night sweats.
  - Symptoms suggestive of an underlying cause, such as hyperthyroidism or pheochromocytoma (e.g., weight loss, palpitations, or persistent fatigue).

## QUESTIONS:

1. **What are the classifications of hyperhidrosis?**
   - Primary Hyperhidrosis and Secondary Hyperhidrosis
     - **Primary Hidrosis** typically occurs in adolescence or younger with a symmetrical pattern, affecting palms, soles, axillae, and/or the face. This type of hyperhidrosis is triggered by stress/emotions and is not considered a systemic disease.
     - **Secondary Hidrosis** occurs at rest; however, it is also influenced by emotional stress. Various causes including thyroid dysfunction, diabetes, infections, some medications, and malignancy.
2. **What are some red flag signs of hyperhidrosis?**
   - Generalised whole-body sweating or the presence of nocturnal sweats.
   - Onset in adulthood.
   - Systemic symptoms such as weight loss, fever, and palpitations.
3. **What blood tests may you consider?**
   - Although this is typically a clinical diagnosis not requiring any labs, it is useful to consider thyroid function tests, glucose, and a complete blood count, especially if secondary hyperhidrosis is suspected.

# CASE 58

# Stimulant Use Disorder in an Adolescent

## Doctor's Notes

*Patient Details:*

- **Name:** Ahmed
- **Age:** 15
- **Occupation:** High school student
- **Presenting Complaint:** Behavioural changes, hyperactivity, academic decline
- **Setting:** Family Medicine Clinic

## PATIENT'S SIMULATED SCRIPT:

### Opening Statement (from parent):

"Doctor, my son has been acting very strangely. He barely sleeps, is always restless, and gets very angry when we ask him about his studies. His grades have dropped, and we found some pills in his room. We're really worried."

## HISTORY:

- **Onset:** Symptoms have gradually developed over the past few months.
- **Behavioural Changes:** Noticeable increase in hyperactivity, restlessness, and aggression. Stays up late with minimal sleep, speaks rapidly, and appears more irritable.
- **Cognitive/Academic Impact:** Difficulty concentrating, academic decline, defensiveness about school performance.
- **Appetite and Weight:** Loss of appetite and recent weight loss.
- **Lifestyle and Social Factors:**
  - High academic expectations from family and school.
  - Recently socializing with older peers.
  - Parents noticed unusual spending habits, uncertain source of expenses.
- **Possible Substance Use:** Parents found stimulant pills in his school bag, raising concerns about non-prescribed medication use.

## DRUG HISTORY:

- **Regular Medications:** None
- **Allergies:** None known
- **Recent Treatments:** No prescribed medications, but suspected unsupervised use of stimulants.

## FAMILY HISTORY:

- No history of psychiatric illness or substance abuse reported.

## IDEAS, CONCERNS, EXPECTATIONS:

- **Ideas:** Parents suspect Ahmed is taking pills to help with studying and academic performance.
- **Concerns:** Fear of developing addiction and long-term health issues.
- **Expectations:** Hoping to understand the cause of his behavioural changes and find appropriate treatment.

## ON EXAMINATION:

- **General Appearance:** Thin, restless, avoids direct eye contact.
- **Vitals:** BP 140/90 mmHg, HR 110 bpm (tachycardic).
- **Neurological Exam:** No focal neurological deficits; fine tremors noted.
- **Mental State Examination:**
    - **Mood:** Anxious and irritable.
    - **Speech:** Pressured.
    - **Thought Process:** Logical, but racing thoughts.
    - **Perception:** No hallucinations, mild paranoia ("feels watched").

## INVESTIGATIONS:

1. **Urine Drug Screen:**
    - Positive for amphetamines/stimulants
    - Negative for THC, opioids, benzodiazepines, cocaine
2. **Blood Tests (CBC, LFTs, Renal Panel):** Normal
3. **ECG:** Mild tachycardia, no arrhythmias
4. **Psychological Screening:**
    - Elevated stress levels linked to academic pressure
    - No current signs of major depressive disorder, but at-risk profile

## WHAT IS THE DIAGNOSIS?

1. **Stimulant Use Disorder** – Likely misuse of prescription stimulants (e.g., Adderall/Ritalin) for cognitive enhancement and academic performance.
2. **Substance-Induced Anxiety Symptoms** – Likely contributing to current behavioural and psychological state.

Stimulant misuse in adolescents is increasingly prevalent, often linked to academic pressures and social influences. Effects include irritability, insomnia, appetite suppression, anxiety, and cardiovascular strain.

## OUTLINE THE MANAGEMENT OPTIONS:

1. **Non-Judgmental Communication:**
   - Create a safe space for the patient to speak openly.
   - Explore reasons behind stimulant use – academic stress? Peer influence?
   - Educate on the medical risks of stimulant misuse (e.g., cardiac complications, mood instability, dependence).
2. **Parental Support and Family Counselling:**
   - Encourage a supportive, non-punitive home environment.
   - Discuss strategies for reducing academic pressure.
   - Promote open communication and realistic expectations.
3. **Medical Management of Withdrawal:**
   - Monitor closely for withdrawal symptoms (fatigue, mood swings, cravings).
   - Encourage regular meals, hydration, and sleep hygiene.
   - Consider gradual tapering under medical supervision if needed.
4. **Mental Health and Behavioural Therapy:**
   - Refer to psychologist for cognitive behavioural therapy (CBT).
   - Teach stress management, goal-setting, and healthy study techniques.
   - Encourage participation in physical activity and hobbies.
5. **Ongoing Monitoring and Follow-up:**
   - Schedule regular follow-ups every 1–2 weeks initially.
   - Repeat urine drug screens if clinically indicated.
   - Monitor for mental health deterioration or risk of relapse.

## FOLLOW-UP AND SAFETY NETTING:

- **Follow-up Plan:**
  - Initial review in 1–2 weeks, then as clinically needed.
  - Reassess progress, adherence to therapy, and home dynamics.
- **Red Flags:**
  - Chest pain, palpitations, or panic attacks.
  - Suicidal ideation or escalating aggression.
  - Severe withdrawal symptoms such as extreme fatigue or depression.
- **Resources:**
  - Adolescent mental health services and substance use support groups.
  - Educational materials for families on managing stimulant misuse.

## QUESTIONS:

1. **What are some commonly recognised complications of adolescent stimulant misuse?**
   - **Cardiovascular:** Tachycardia, hypertension, arrhythmias, and in rare cases cardiac arrest.
   - **Psychiatric:** Anxiety, agitation, paranoid thoughts, labile mood, depression and/or psychosis.
   - **Neurological:** Memory deficits, poor attention and general academic decline.
   - **Social:** Risk-taking behaviour, family conflict, and peer influence.
2. **What clinical features suggest stimulant misuse?**
   - Hyperactivity, restlessness, irritability, aggression.
   - Insomnia, reduced appetite, weight loss.
   - Rapid speech, racing thoughts, mild paranoia.
   - Tremors, tachycardia, hypertension.
   - Academic decline, social withdrawal, or secrecy.

# CASE 59 Growing Pains

## Doctor's Notes

*Patient Details:*

- **Name:** Sarah Hassan
- **Age:** 7
- **Occupation:** Primary school student
- **Presenting Complaint:** Intermittent leg pain, mostly at night
- **Setting:** Family Medicine Clinic

## PATIENT'S SIMULATED SCRIPT:

### Opening Statement (parent):

"Doctor, my daughter has been waking up at night with leg pain. It's been happening for a few months now. Is this something serious?"

## HISTORY:

- **Onset and Duration:** Intermittent leg pain for the past few months.
- **Timing:** Typically occurs at night, often wakes the child from sleep; resolves by morning.
- **Location:** Bilateral pain affecting the thighs and calves.
- **Character:** Dull ache, non-localized.
- **Associated Symptoms:** No redness, swelling, warmth, or stiffness. No trauma.
- **Pattern:** No daytime pain, no limping, and full activity maintained during the day.
- **Impact:** Occasionally disrupts sleep, requiring comfort from parents.

## LIFESTYLE AND RISK FACTORS:

- Active and playful during the day.
- Diet a mix of home-cooked and processed food.
- No known nutritional deficiencies, though sun exposure is limited.

## ATTEMPTS TO MANAGE:

- Parents have tried gentle massage and warm compresses with temporary relief.
- No medications given prior to consultation.

## DRUG HISTORY:

- **Regular Medications:** None
- **Allergies:** None known

## FAMILY HISTORY:

- No known autoimmune or metabolic bone conditions.
- Father recalls similar symptoms during his childhood.

## IDEAS, CONCERNS, EXPECTATIONS:

- **Ideas:** Parents suspect it might be arthritis or a more serious bone disorder.
- **Concerns:** That the pain might affect growth or mobility.
- **Expectations:** Looking for reassurance and guidance on how to manage or prevent further episodes.

## ON EXAMINATION:

- **General Appearance:** Alert, well-nourished, and interactive.
- **Vital Signs:** BP 98/62 mmHg, HR 92 bpm, Temp 36.7°C
- **Musculoskeletal Exam:**
  - No joint tenderness, swelling, or warmth.
  - Full range of motion in all joints.
  - No gait abnormality or signs of muscle weakness.
  - No limb length discrepancy.

## INVESTIGATIONS AND RESULTS:

1. **Blood Tests:**
   - **Calcium:** Normal
   - **Vitamin D:** Slightly low (20 ng/mL)
   - **CBC, CRP, ESR:** All within normal limits
2. **Imaging:**
   - **X-ray of lower limbs:** Normal bone development, no fractures or abnormalities.

## DIAGNOSIS:

1. **Growing Pains (benign nocturnal limb pains of childhood).**
2. **Mild Vitamin D Deficiency.**

Growing pains are benign, self-limiting episodes of musculoskeletal pain common in children aged 3–12 years. Although the exact cause is unknown, it may relate to increased activity levels and muscle fatigue. Importantly, they do not impair growth or joint function.

## OUTLINE THE MANAGEMENT OPTIONS:

1. **Parental Reassurance:**
   - Emphasize that the condition is common and not associated with any serious illness or growth disorder.
   - Educate on the benign and self-limiting nature of the symptoms.
2. **Symptom Management:**
   - Leg massage before bed.
   - Warm compresses during painful episodes.
   - Paracetamol or ibuprofen during severe pain episodes (not routinely needed).
   - Gentle stretching before bedtime.
3. **Address Vitamin D Deficiency:**
   - Start vitamin D supplementation (400–600 IU daily).
   - Encourage increased sun exposure and consumption of vitamin D–rich foods.
4. **Lifestyle Measures:**
   - Balanced diet with adequate calcium.
   - Encourage physical activity while avoiding overexertion.

## FOLLOW-UP AND SAFETY NETTING:

- **Review Plan:**
  - Follow-up in 6–8 weeks to assess symptom improvement.
  - Recheck vitamin D levels after 3 months if symptoms persist.
- **Red Flags to Watch For:**
  - Daytime pain or persistent limp.
  - Swelling or redness of joints.
  - Unexplained fever, weight loss, or fatigue.
  - Neurological symptoms or significant weakness.

## QUESTIONS

1. **What are red flag signs that would suggest a different diagnosis?**
   - Ongoing persistent pain or limping
   - Swelling, redness, and pain in joints
   - Systemic symptoms (fever, weight loss, fatigue)
   - Numbness or gait abnormalities
2. **What is the pathophysiology of this condition?**
   - Exact cause unknown; however, it is thought to be related to a number of factors:
     - Muscle soreness and fatigue at the end of a day of high activity.
     - Lower pain thresholds.
     - Musculoskeletal factors (flat feet, joint hypermobility).
     - Emotional factors, thought to play a role in triggering or exacerbating pain in children.
3. **What is the differential diagnosis for intermittent nocturnal leg pain in children?**
   - Juvenile idiopathic arthritis.
   - Osteomyelitis or bone infection.
   - Trauma/fracture.
   - Osteoid osteoma.
   - Benign tumours or malignancy (rare).
   - Vitamin D deficiency–related bone pain.

# CASE 60
# Missed Vaccinations

## Doctor's Notes

*Patient Details:*

- **Name:** Noah Thompson
- **Age:** 18 months
- **Occupation:** N/A
- **Presenting Complaint:** Parents seeking advice about missed vaccinations
- **Setting:** Family Medicine Clinic

## PATIENT'S SIMULATED SCRIPT:

### Opening Statement:

"Doctor, we missed Noah's last vaccination appointment, and we're worried if that's going to be a problem."

## HISTORY:

- **Current History:**
  - **Immunization Status:** Up to date until the 12-month vaccines but missed the 18-month vaccines due to travel.
  - **Reason for Delay:** Family was abroad visiting relatives and missed the scheduled appointment.
  - **Parents' Concerns:** Worried about the risks of delayed vaccines and potential catch-up schedules.
  - **Adverse Reactions:** No previous allergic reactions or complications from previous immunizations.
- **Drug History:**
  - **Regular Medications:** None.
  - **Allergies:** None known.
- **Family History:**
  - No family history of immune disorders or vaccine-related issues.

## IDEAS, CONCERNS, EXPECTATIONS:

- **Ideas:** Parents understand that vaccines are important but are unsure if a delay can affect effectiveness.
- **Concerns:** Worried that the delay might leave Noah vulnerable to diseases or that they might have missed the opportunity to catch up.
- **Expectations:** Looking for reassurance that Noah can still receive the missed vaccines without long-term effects.

## ON EXAMINATION:

- **General Appearance:** Healthy, alert, and well-nourished toddler.
- **Vital Signs:** Normal and age-appropriate.
- **Growth and Development:** Meeting age-appropriate milestones.

## WHAT IS THE DIAGNOSIS?

**Delayed Immunization** – routine catch-up needed.

Missing a scheduled vaccine dose is not uncommon, and catch-up immunization is typically straightforward. Timely vaccinations are essential to protect children from preventable diseases, but catch-up schedules ensure that children remain protected even if doses are delayed.

## OUTLINE THE MANAGEMENT OPTIONS:

1. **Catch-up Immunization:**
   - Administer the missed 18-month vaccines today, including the DTaP/IPV/Hib booster and MMR if not received at 12 months.
   - Ensure the next scheduled vaccines are booked to prevent further delays.
2. **Reassurance:**
   - Explain that a short delay does not reduce vaccine effectiveness.
   - Emphasize that it is never too late to catch up and that completing the series provides full protection.
3. **Education:**
   - Highlight the importance of staying on schedule to prevent diseases like measles, polio, and whooping cough.
   - Provide a written immunization schedule and discuss the next vaccination at 4 years.
4. **Red Flags:**
   - Advise parents to monitor for common side effects such as mild fever, redness, or swelling at the injection site.
   - Seek medical advice if severe allergic reactions (rash, difficulty breathing) occur, though these are rare.

## QUESTIONS:

1. **Are there any risks associated with delayed vaccinations?**
   - Child may remain temporarily susceptible to certain infections until doses are given.
   - Increased risk of infection only during the unvaccinated period.
2. **What is the recommended approach for a child with missed vaccines?**
   - Catch up with immunizations and administer the missed doses without restarting the schedule.
   - Maintain the minimum intervals between doses – this allows for establishing proper immunity.

# CASE 61 Constipation

## Doctor's Notes

*Patient Details:*

- **Name:** Zahra Ali
- **Age:** 4 years
- **Occupation:** N/A
- **Presenting Complaint:** Constipation for the past 2 weeks
- **Setting:** Family Medicine Clinic

## PATIENT'S SIMULATED SCRIPT:

### Opening Statement:

"Doctor, Zahra hasn't been able to go to the toilet properly for the last 2 weeks."

## HISTORY:

- **Onset:** Started 2 weeks ago, with bowel movements becoming less frequent.
- **Frequency:** Passing stools every 3–4 days, hard and pellet-like.
- **Associated Symptoms:** Occasional abdominal discomfort, straining during bowel movements, no blood in the stool, and no vomiting.
- **Dietary History:** Prefers processed foods, low intake of fruits and vegetables, and drinks minimal water.
- **Toilet Training:** Recently started toilet training, causing some anxiety and reluctance to use the toilet.
- **Previous Episodes:** Occasional constipation in the past, but this is the longest episode.

## DRUG HISTORY:

- **Regular Medications:** None.
- **Allergies:** None known.

## FAMILY HISTORY:

- No family history of gastrointestinal disorders.

## IDEAS, CONCERNS, EXPECTATIONS:

- **Ideas:** Parents think Zahra's constipation might be due to her diet and toilet training.
- **Concerns:** Worried that prolonged constipation could cause long-term problems or lead to pain and fear of using the toilet.
- **Expectations:** Seeking advice on relieving constipation and preventing it from recurring.

## ON EXAMINATION:

- **General Appearance:** Healthy, alert, and active child.
- **Vitals:** Normal and age-appropriate.
- **Abdominal Examination:** Mild distension, no tenderness or guarding, palpable stool in the lower abdomen, normal bowel sounds.

## WHAT IS THE DIAGNOSIS:

**Functional Constipation.**

This is common in young children, often related to dietary factors, toilet training, or withholding behaviour. Timely management is essential to prevent chronic constipation and associated complications.

## OUTLINE THE MANAGEMENT OPTIONS:

1. **Dietary Modifications:**
   - Increase fibre intake through fruits (e.g., apples, pears, berries), vegetables, and whole grains.
   - Encourage adequate water intake to soften stools.
   - Limit processed foods, dairy products, and sugary snacks.
2. **Behavioural Interventions:**
   - Establish a regular toilet routine, encouraging Zahra to sit on the toilet after meals (gastrocolic reflex) without pressure or punishment.
   - Use positive reinforcement (praise, stickers) to encourage toilet use.
3. **Medications:**
   - Prescribe a gentle laxative (e.g., polyethylene glycol or lactulose) to soften stools and reduce straining.
   - Avoid stimulant laxatives unless necessary.
4. **Parental Education:**
   - Explain that constipation is common and treatable, with no long-term effects if managed promptly.
   - Emphasize patience and consistency in dietary and toilet habits.

## RED FLAGS (IF PRESENT; REQUIRE FURTHER INVESTIGATION):

- Persistent constipation despite treatment.
- Blood in the stool, weight loss, or failure to thrive.
- Vomiting, abdominal distension, or severe pain.

## FOLLOW-UP:

- Review progress in 2 weeks to assess stool frequency and consistency.
- Adjust laxative dosage if needed, ensuring stools remain soft and easy to pass.

## QUESTIONS:

1. **What are the signs that would suggest an organic cause?**
   - Blood in the stool
   - Failure to thrive/weight loss (non-intentional)
   - Limb weakness or abnormal reflexes
   - Signs systemic illness
2. **What initial investigations are recommended for functional constipation?** (only if diagnostic uncertainty/presence of red flags)
   - Abdominal x-ray (to investigate faecal loading or impaction)
   - Labs: CBC, thyroid panel, electrolytes (when suspecting systemic illness)
   - Coeliac screen when growth issues or chronic diarrhoea
3. **What complications can occur if constipation is not managed?**
   - Faecal impaction
   - Overflow diarrhoea
   - Painful defecation
   - Anal fissures
   - Urinary retention

CASE

# 62

# Seasonal Affective Disorder

## Doctor's Notes

*Patient Details:*

- **Name:** Omar A.
- **Age:** 30
- **Occupation:** Software Developer
- **Presenting Complaint:** Low energy, poor concentration, and low motivation for the past few winters
- **Setting:** Family Medicine Clinic

## PATIENT'S SIMULATED SCRIPT:

### Opening Statement:

"Doctor, I just can't seem to get back into the rhythm of things. I feel off."

## HISTORY OF PRESENTING ILLNESS:

- **Onset:** Symptoms began approximately three winters ago, recurring annually.
- **Duration:** Each episode lasts from late fall to early spring (around 4–5 months).
- **Symptoms:**
  - Fatigue and low motivation
  - Difficulty concentrating
  - Oversleeping (up to 10 hours/day)
  - Increased carbohydrate cravings and mild weight gain
  - Low mood and flat affect during winter months
  - No suicidal ideation or feelings of worthlessness
  - Describes himself as "in a fog" during the winter; mood improves significantly in summer
- **Contextual Factors:**
  - Relocated from UAE to Sweden 3 years ago for work
  - Reports decreased sun exposure and outdoor activity since moving
- **Previous Episodes:** None before relocation

- **Impact on Function:** Struggles with productivity and socializing in winter
- **No symptoms of mania or psychosis**
- **No prior psychiatric diagnoses**

## PAST MEDICAL HISTORY:

- No chronic medical conditions
- No psychiatric history

## DRUG HISTORY:

- Takes multivitamins occasionally
- No regular medications
- No known allergies

## FAMILY HISTORY:

- Mother has type 2 diabetes
- No known family history of mood disorders

## SOCIAL HISTORY:

- Lives alone
- Alternates between remote and in-office work
- Minimal physical activity and limited sunlight exposure in winter
- No tobacco, alcohol, or drug use

## REVIEW OF SYSTEMS:

- No appetite loss or major anxiety
- No suicidal thoughts
- No manic symptoms

## MENTAL STATE EXAMINATION:

- **Appearance:** Casual, slightly dishevelled
- **Speech:** Normal
- **Mood:** Flat
- **Affect:** Restricted
- **Thoughts:** No delusions, no suicidal ideation
- **Cognition:** Mild difficulties with attention
- **Insight:** Fair

## IDEAS, CONCERNS, EXPECTATIONS:

- **Ideas:** Omar believes his symptoms could be "burnout" or weather-related.
- **Concerns:** Worried that this is becoming a yearly pattern and might worsen over time.
- **Expectations:** Hopes for an explanation and tools to manage or prevent these symptoms.

## WHAT IS THE DIAGNOSIS AND DIFFERENTIAL DIAGNOSIS?

1. **Seasonal Affective Disorder (SAD)** – Most likely, given clear seasonal pattern, atypical depressive features (hypersomnia, carb cravings).

2. **Persistent Depressive Disorder** (less likely due to symptom-free periods).
3. **Hypothyroidism** (must be excluded).
4. **Burnout or Adjustment Disorder** (though seasonal consistency makes SAD more likely).

## RED FLAGS TO CONSIDER:

- Active suicidal ideation
- Functional impairment affecting daily living or work
- Psychotic features
- Past manic episodes (rule out bipolar disorder)
- Weight loss, insomnia (non-atypical depression signs)

## INVESTIGATIONS:

1. **TSH, Free T4:** Rule out hypothyroidism
2. **CBC, Vitamin D:** Screen for anaemia or deficiencies
3. **PHQ-9 or other depression scales:** To quantify severity
4. **Mood diary or seasonal pattern chart:** For confirming temporal trends

## OUTLINE THE MANAGEMENT PLAN:

1. **Lifestyle Modifications:**
   - Encourage daily morning exposure to natural light or light therapy (10,000 lux) for 30 minutes/day
   - Promote regular physical activity, ideally outdoors
   - Minimize carbohydrate-heavy snacking
2. **Psychological Support:**
   - Consider referral for cognitive behavioural therapy (CBT), especially CBT-SAD (seasonal variant)
   - Monitor for mood changes across seasons
3. **Pharmacotherapy (if moderate-severe):**
   - Discuss potential benefits of initiating an SSRI during high-risk months (e.g., sertraline)
   - Consider bupropion XL, which has some evidence for SAD prevention
4. **Patient Education:**
   - Explain that SAD is a recognized subtype of depression with a seasonal pattern
   - Reassure that it is manageable with consistent treatment and awareness

## SAFETY NETTING:

- Advise Omar to seek immediate help if he develops suicidal thoughts or significant functional decline
- Provide mental health crisis contacts
- Encourage maintaining a mood diary to track patterns over time

## QUESTIONS:

1. **What investigations can you consider when diagnosing SAD?**
   - Thyroid function panel (in case hypothyroid)
   - CBC, Vitamin D – being anaemic or deficient in vitamin D can worsen fatigue/mood
   - Depression severity scores (PHQ-9s)
   - Mood diary
2. **How should follow-up be arranged?**
   - Review in 2–3 weeks to assess response to non-pharmacological interventions
   - Monitor the mood, sleep, and general daily functioning
   - Refer to psychiatry if the patient deteriorates

# CASE 63

# Fasting in Ramadan, the Hypertensive Type 2 Diabetic

## Doctor's Notes

*Patient Details:*

- **Name:** Faisal Al-Mansoori
- **Age:** 52
- **Gender:** Male
- **Occupation:** Accountant
- **Presenting Complaint:** Advice regarding fasting during Ramadan
- **Setting:** Family Medicine Clinic

## PATIENT'S SIMULATED SCRIPT:

### Opening Statement:

"Assalamu Alaykom (Peace be upon you), Doctor! Ramadan is starting next week and I am concerned, as I take medications for my blood pressure and diabetes. Can I fast safely?"

## HISTORY:

- **History of Presenting Complaint:**
  - **Diabetes:** Diagnosed 8 years ago; currently on metformin 1 g twice daily and gliclazide 80 mg once daily.
  - **Hypertension:** Diagnosed 5 years ago; currently on amlodipine 5 mg daily and losartan 50 mg daily.
  - **Fasting History:** Fasted in previous years; experienced mild dizziness and one episode of hypoglycaemia last year.
  - **Symptoms:** No current hypoglycaemia, no syncope, no chest pain.
- **Past Medical History:**
  - Type 2 diabetes mellitus, well-controlled (HbA1c 7.2%)
  - Hypertension, controlled
- **Drug History:**
  - Metformin 1 g BID
  - Gliclazide 80 mg OD

  - Amlodipine 5 mg OD
  - Losartan 50 mg OD
  - No allergies
- **Lifestyle and Social History:**
  - Non-smoker, no alcohol
  - Sedentary office work, walks 30 minutes 3×/week
  - Eats regular meals, avoids skipping meals
- **Family History:**
  - Father – hypertension and type 2 diabetes mellitus
  - Mother – type 2 diabetes

## IDEAS, CONCERNS, EXPECTATIONS:

- **Ideas:** Worried fasting might worsen blood sugar or blood pressure.
- **Concerns:** Hypoglycemia or hypotension while fasting.
- **Expectations:** Wants to fast safely without complications.

## EXAMINATION:

- **General Appearance:** Well, alert
- **Vital Signs:** BP 128/82 mmHg, HR 78 bpm, temperature 36.7°C
- **Weight:** 82 kg, BMI 28
- **Other Systems:** Normal; no dehydration, hypoglycaemia signs, or cardiovascular compromise

## INVESTIGATIONS:

- **Fasting Blood Glucose:** 110 mg/dL
- **HbA1c:** 7.2%
- **Renal Function and Electrolytes:** Normal

## KNOWN DIAGNOSIS:

1. **Type 2 Diabetes Mellitus,** stable.
2. **Hypertension,** controlled.

## OUTLINE THE MANAGEMENT PLAN:

1. **Medication Adjustments:**
   - **Metformin:** Continue; shift doses to Suhoor and Iftar (split 500 mg at Suhoor, 500 mg at Iftar).
   - **Gliclazide → Sitagliptin:** Replace sulfonylurea with Sitagliptin 100 mg once daily at Suhoor or Iftar.
     - Reason: Low risk of hypoglycemia, safer for fasting.
   - **Amlodipine and Losartan:** Continue, take at Iftar to avoid hypotension while fasting.
2. **Lifestyle and Diet:**
   - Maintain balanced meals at Suhoor and Iftar.
   - Avoid excessive sugary foods at Iftar.
   - Stay hydrated between Iftar and Suhoor.
   - Moderate physical activity after Iftar.

3. **Monitoring and Safety Netting:**
   - Monitor blood glucose at Suhoor, mid-day (if feasible), and Iftar initially.
   - Break fast if:
     - **Blood glucose <70 mg/dL** (hypoglycaemia)
     - **Blood glucose >300 mg/dL** (hyperglycaemia)
     - Dizziness, syncope, severe thirst, or palpitations
4. **Patient Education:**
   - Explain the risk of hypoglycaemia with sulfonylureas.
   - Discuss importance of medication timing and meal planning.
   - Emphasize when to stop fasting safely.
5. **Follow-up:**
   - Review 1–2 weeks after Ramadan starts to monitor symptoms, blood glucose, and blood pressure.
   - Adjust medications if required.

## QUESTIONS:

1. **What are the main risks for patients with diabetes fasting during Ramadan?**
   - Hypoglycaemia (especially on sulfonylureas or insulin)
   - Hyperglycaemia (missed meals, overeating at Iftar)
   - Dehydration, hypotension
   - Thrombosis risk (if poorly hydrated)
   - Exacerbation of comorbid conditions (renal or cardiovascular)
2. **How can we reduce the hypoglycaemia risk for this patient?**
   - Replace sulfonylureas with DPP-4 inhibitors (sitagliptin) or other low-risk medications
   - Adjust timing of medications at Suhoor and Iftar
   - Monitor blood glucose regularly
   - Educate patient to break the fast if symptomatic hypoglycemia occurs
3. **Do we need to make any adjustments to the blood pressure medication?**
   - Take antihypertensives at Iftar to reduce risk of hypotension while fasting
   - Continue usual doses if blood pressure is stable
   - Monitor for dizziness or syncope

www.ingramcontent.com/pod-product-compliance
Lightning Source LLC
LaVergne TN
LVHW080039210926
848481LV00011B/3238

* 9 7 8 1 2 6 5 7 8 5 7 2 7 *